This report contains the collective views of an international group of experts and does not necessarily represent the decisions or the stated policy of the United Nations Environment Programme, the International Labour Organisation, or the World Health Organization.

Environmental Health Criteria 123

ALPHA- AND BETA-HEXACHLOROCYCLOHEXANES

First draft prepared by Dr G.J. van Esch, Bilthoven, The Netherlands

Published under the joint sponsorship of the United Nations Environment Programme, the International Labour Organisation, and the World Health Organization

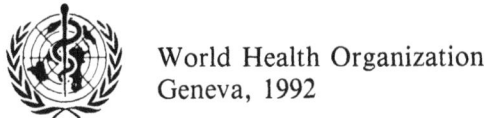

World Health Organization
Geneva, 1992

The **International Programme on Chemical Safety** (IPCS) is a joint venture of the United Nations Environment Programme, the International Labour Organisation, and the World Health Organization. The main objective of the IPCS is to carry out and disseminate evaluations of the effects of chemicals on human health and the quality of the environment. Supporting activities include the development of epidemiological, experimental laboratory, and risk-assessment methods that could produce internationally comparable results, and the development of manpower in the field of toxicology. Other activities carried out by the IPCS include the development of know-how for coping with chemical accidents, coordination of laboratory testing and epidemiological studies, and promotion of research on the mechanisms of the biological action of chemicals.

WHO Library Cataloguing in Publication Data

Alpha- and beta-hexachlorocyclohexanes.

(Environmental health criteria ; 123)

1.Benzene hexachloride - adverse effects 2.Benzene hexachloride - toxicity 3.Environmental exposure 4.Environmental pollutants I.Series

ISBN 92 4 157123 3   (NLM Classification: QV 633)
ISSN 0250-863X

©World Health Organization 1991

Publications of the World Health Organization enjoy copyright protection in accordance with the provisions of Protocol 2 of the Universal Copyright Convention. For rights of reproduction or translation of WHO publications, in part or *in toto,* application should be made to the Office of Publications, World Health Organization, Geneva, Switzerland. The World Health Organization welcomes such applications.

The designations employed and the presentation of the material in this publication do not imply the expression of any opinion whatsoever on the part of the Secretariat of the World Health Organization concerning the legal status of any country, territory, city, or area or of its authorities, or concerning the delimitation of its frontiers or boundaries.

The mention of specific companies or of certain manufacturers' products does not imply that they are endorsed or recommended by the World Health Organization in preference to others of a similar nature that are not mentioned. Errors and omissions excepted, the names of proprietary products are distinguished by initial capital letters.

Printed in Finland
92/9020 — Vammala — 5500

CONTENTS

ENVIRONMENTAL HEALTH CRITERIA FOR
ALPHA- AND BETA-HEXACHLOROCYCLOHEXANES

A. ALPHA-HEXACHLOROCYCLOHEXANE	9
B. BETA-HEXACHLOROCYCLOHEXANE	67
CONCLUSIONS AND RECOMMENDATIONS FOR PROTECTION OF HUMAN HEALTH AND THE ENVIRONMENT (ALPHA- AND BETA-HEXACHLOROCYCLOHEXANES)	118
FURTHER RESEARCH (ALPHA- AND BETA-HEXACHLOROCYCLOHEXANES)	120
PREVIOUS EVALUATIONS BY INTERNATIONAL BODIES	121
REFERENCES	122
APPENDIX 1. CHEMICAL STRUCTURE	140

RESUME ET EVALUATION

1. Alpha-hexachlorocyclohexane	141
2. Béta-hexachlorocyclohexane	147
CONCLUSIONS ET RECOMMANDATIONS	153
RECHERCHES A EFFECTUER (ALPHA- ET BETA-HEXACHLOROCYCLOHEXANES)	155

RESUMEN Y EVALUACION

1. Alpha-hexaclorociclohexano	156
2. Beta-hexaclorociclohexano	162
CONCLUSIONES Y RECOMENDACIONES	168
OTRAS INVESTIGACIONES (ALPHA- Y BETA-HEXACLOROCICLOHEXANOS)	170

WHO TASK GROUP MEETING ON ENVIRONMENTAL HEALTH CRITERIA FOR ALPHA- AND BETA-HEXACHLOROCYCLOHEXANES

Members

Dr S. Dobson, Institute of Terrestrial Ecology, Monkswood Experimental Station, Abbots Ripton, Huntingdon, United Kingdom

Dr M. Herbst, ASTA Pharma A.G., Frankfurt, Germany *(Joint Rapporteur)*

Professor J.S. Kagan, Department of General Toxicology and Experimental Pathology, All-Union Scientific Research Institute of Hygiene and Toxicology of Pesticides, Polymers, and Plastics, Kiev, USSR *(Vice-Chairman)*

Dr S.G.A. Magwood, Pesticides Division, Environmental Health Centre, Health & Welfare Canada, Tunney's Pasture, Ottawa, Ontario, Canada

Professor Wai-On Phoon, National Institute of Occupational Health and Safety, University of Sydney, Sydney, Australia *(Chairman)*

Dr J.F. Risher, US Environmental Protection Agency, Environmental Criteria and Assessment Office, Cincinnati, Ohio, USA

Dr Y. Saito, Division of Foods, National Institute of Hygienic Sciences, Setagaya-ku, Tokyo, Japan

Dr V. Turusov, Laboratory of Carcinogenic Substances, All-Union Cancer Research Centre, Moscow, USSR

Dr G.J. van Esch, Bilthoven, The Netherlands *(Joint Rapporteur)*

Representatives of Non-Governmental Organizations

Dr P.G. Pontal, International Group of National Associations of Manufacturers of Agrochemical Products (GIFAP), Rhône-Poulenc Agro, Lyon, France

Observers

Dr A.V. Bolotny, All-Union Scientific Research Institute of Hygiene and Toxicology of Pesticides, Polymers, and Plastics, Kiev, USSR

Dr D. Demozay, International Centre for Study on Lindane (CIEL), Rhône-Poulenc Agro, Lyon, France

Secretariat

Dr G.J. Burin, International Programme on Chemical Safety, World Health Organization, Geneva, Switzerland

Dr K.W. Jager, International Programme on Chemical Safety, World Health Organization, Geneva, Switzerland *(Secretary)*

Dr V.A. Rezepov, Centre for International Projects, USSR State Committee for Environmental Protection, Moscow, USSR

NOTE TO READERS OF THE CRITERIA MONOGRAPHS

Every effort has been made to present information in the criteria monographs as accurately as possible without unduly delaying their publication. In the interest of all users of the environmental health criteria monographs, readers are kindly requested to communicate any errors that may have occurred to the Manager of the International Programme on Chemical Safety, World Health Organization, Geneva, Switzerland, in order that they may be included in corrigenda.

* * *

A detailed data profile and a legal file can be obtained from the International Register of Potentially Toxic Chemicals, Palais des Nations, 1211 Geneva 10, Switzerland (Telephone No. 7988400 or 7985850).

ENVIRONMENTAL HEALTH CRITERIA FOR ALPHA- AND BETA-HEXACHLOROCYCLOHEXANES

A WHO Task Group on Environmental Health Criteria for Alpha- and Beta-hexachlorocyclohexanes met in Moscow from 20 to 24 November 1989. The meeting was convened with the financial assistance of the United Nations Environment Programme (UNEP) and was hosted by the Centre for International Projects (CIP), USSR State Committee for Environmental Protection. Dr V.A. Rezepov opened the meeting on behalf of the CIP and welcomed the participants. Dr K.W. Jager welcomed the participants on behalf of the three IPCS cooperating organizations (UNEP/ILO/WHO). The Task Group reviewed and revised the draft criteria monograph and made an evaluation of the risks for human health and the environment from exposure to alpha- and beta-hexachlorocyclohexanes.

The first and second drafts of this monograph were prepared by Dr G.J. van Esch (on behalf of the IPCS). Dr K.W. Jager and Dr P.G. Jenkins, both members of the IPCS Central Unit, were responsible for the overall scientific content and technical editing, respectively.

The efforts of all who helped in the preparation and finalization of the document are gratefully acknowledged.

ABBREVIATIONS

cGMP	cyclic guanosine monophosphate
CNS	central nervous system
EEG	electroencephalogram
EMG	electromyogram
FDA	Food and Drug Administration (USA)
FSH	follicle-stimulating hormone
GABA	gamma-aminobutyric acid
GGT	gamma-glutamyltransferase
GLC	gas-liquid chromatography
HCB	hexachlorobenzene
HCCH	hexachlorocyclohexene
HCH	hexachlorocyclohexane
ip	intraperitoneal
LH	luteinizing hormone
MTD	maximum tolerated dose
nd	not detected
NOEL	no-observed-effect level
PCB	polychlorinated biphenyl
PCCH	pentachlorocyclohexane
PIC	picrotoxin
PTZ	pentylenetetrazole
SEM	smooth endoplasmic reticulum

PART A

ENVIRONMENTAL HEALTH CRITERIA

FOR

ALPHA-HEXACHLOROCYCLOHEXANE

CONTENTS

ENVIRONMENTAL HEALTH CRITERIA FOR
ALPHA-HEXACHLOROCYCLOHEXANE

1. SUMMARY AND EVALUATION   13

    1.1 General properties   13
    1.2 Environmental transport, distribution, and
         transformation   13
    1.3 Environmental levels and human exposure   13
    1.4 Kinetics and metabolism   15
    1.5 Effects on organisms in the environment   15
    1.6 Effects on experimental animals and
         in vitro test systems   16
    1.7 Effects on humans   17

2. IDENTITY, PHYSICAL AND CHEMICAL
   PROPERTIES, ANALYTICAL METHODS   18

    2.1 Identity of primary constituent   18
    2.2 Physical and chemical properties   18
    2.3 Analytical methods   19

3. SOURCES OF HUMAN AND ENVIRONMENTAL
   EXPOSURE   20

4. ENVIRONMENTAL TRANSPORT, DISTRIBUTION,
   AND TRANSFORMATION   21

    4.1 Transport and distribution between media   21
    4.2 Biotransformation   22
         4.2.1 Biodegradation   22
         4.2.2 Abiotic degradation   24
         4.2.3 Bioaccumulation/biomagnification   24
                4.2.3.1 Algae   24
                4.2.3.2 Invertebrates   25
                4.2.3.3 Fish   25
                4.2.3.4 Bioconcentration in humans   27
    4.3 Isomerization   28

5. ENVIRONMENTAL LEVELS AND HUMAN EXPOSURE 29

5.1 Environmental levels 29
    5.1.1 Air 29
    5.1.2 Water 29
        5.1.2.1 Rain water 29
        5.1.2.2 Fresh water 30
        5.1.2.3 Sea water 31
    5.1.3 Soil/sediment 31
        5.1.3.1 Dumping grounds 32
    5.1.4 Food and feed 32
    5.1.5 Terrestrial and aquatic organisms 35
        5.1.5.1 Plants 35
        5.1.5.2 Fish and mussels 35
        5.1.5.3 Birds 36
        5.1.5.4 Mammals 37
5.2 General population exposure 38
    5.2.1 Total-diet studies 38
    5.2.2 Air 39
    5.2.3 Concentrations in human samples 39
        5.2.3.1 Blood 39
        5.2.3.2 Adipose tissue 40
        5.2.3.3 Breast milk 41

6. KINETICS AND METABOLISM 43

6.1 Absorption and elimination 43
6.2 Distribution 43
6.3 Metabolic transformation 44
    6.3.1 Rat 44
    6.3.2 Bird 45
    6.3.3 Human 45
6.4 Retention and biological half-life 46

7. EFFECTS ON LABORATORY MAMMALS AND
   IN VITRO TEST SYSTEMS 47

7.1 Single exposure 47
    7.1.1 Acute toxicity 47
7.2 Short-term exposure 47
    7.2.1 Oral 47
    7.2.2 Other routes 48
        7.2.2.1 Intravenous 48
        7.2.2.2 Subcutaneous 48

7.3	Skin and eye irritation; sensitization	48
7.4	Long-term exposure	48
	7.4.1 Rat oral study	48
7.5	Reproduction, embryotoxicity, and teratogenicity	49
7.6	Mutagenicity and related end-points	49
7.7	Carcinogenicity	49
	7.7.1 Mouse	50
	7.7.2 Rat	52
	7.7.3 Initiation-promotion	53
	7.7.4 Mode of action	55
7.8	Special studies	55
	7.8.1 Effect on liver enzymes	55
	7.8.2 Neurotoxicity	56

8. EFFECTS ON HUMANS 58

8.1	Acute toxicity - poisoning incidents	58
8.2	General population	58
8.3	Occupational exposure	58

9. EFFECTS ON OTHER ORGANISMS IN THE LABORATORY AND FIELD 61

9.1	Algae		61
9.2	Protozoa		61
9.3	Invertebrates		61
	9.3.1 Acute toxicity		61
	9.3.2 Short- and long-term toxicity		63
		9.3.2.1 Crustaceae	63
		9.3.2.2 Molluscs	63
9.4	Fish		65
	9.4.1 Acute toxicity		65
	9.4.2 Short- and long-term toxicity		65
9.5	Terrestrial organisms		65

1. SUMMARY AND EVALUATION

1.1 General properties

Alpha-hexachlorocyclohexane (alpha-HCH) is a by-product (65-70%) in the manufacture of lindane (> 99% gamma-HCH). Its solubility in water is low, but it is very soluble in organic solvents such as acetone, chloroform, and xylene. It is a solid with a low vapour pressure. The n-octanol/water partition coefficient (log P_{ow}) is 3.82. It is an environmental pollutant.

Alpha-HCH can be determined separately from the other isomers by gas chromatography with electron capture detection and other methods after extraction by liquid/liquid partition and purification by column chromatography.

1.2 Environmental transport, distribution, and transformation

Biodegradation and abiotic degradation (dechlorination) by ultraviolet irradiation occur in the environment and produce, respectively, delta-3,4,5,6-tetrachlorohexene and pentachlorocyclohexene. This breakdown process is slower than in the case of lindane. The persistence of alpha-HCH in soil is determined by environmental factors such as the action of microorganisms, organic matter content, and co-distillation and evaporation from soils. No isomerization occurs from lindane to alpha-HCH.

Rapid bioconcentration takes place in microorganisms (the bioconcentration factor equals 1500-2700 on a dry-weight basis, or approximately 12 000 on a lipid basis within 30 min), invertebrates (60-2750 (dry weight basis) or > 8000 (lipid basis) within 24-72 h), and fish (313-1216 within 4-28 days; up to 50 000 in the River Elbe). However, biotransformation and elimination is also fairly rapid in these organisms (15 min to 72 h).

1.3 Environmental levels and human exposure

Alpha-HCH is found in air over the oceans at a concentration of 0.02-1.5 ng/m^3. In Canada, it was found to be present in rain water at a concentration of 1-40 ng/litre, but only traces were present in snow.

Summary and Evaluation

During the period 1969-1974, the River Rhine and its tributaries contained alpha-HCH levels of 0.01-2.7 µg per litre, but more recently the levels have been below 0.1 µg/litre. In the River Elbe, levels decreased from a mean of 0.023 µg/litre in 1981 to below 0.012 µg per litre in 1988. Selected rivers in the United Kingdom were found in 1966 to contain 0.001-0.43 µg/litre. Alpha-HCH has been found in North Frisian Wadden Sea sediment at concentrations of between 0.3 and 1.4 µg/kg (0.002 µg per litre in water).

Alpha-HCH levels in different plant species from various countries varied from 0.5-2140 µg/kg on a dry-weight basis, but were much higher in polluted areas. Even in Antarctica, levels ranging from 0.2-1.15 µg/kg have been found.

Alpha-HCH is regularly detected in fish and aquatic invertebrates, as well as in ducks, herons, and barn-owls. In reindeer and Idaho moose, living in areas with negligible use of pesticides, average amounts of alpha-HCH of approximately 70-80 µg/kg were found in the subcutaneous fat. The adipose tissue of Canadian polar bears contained 0.3-0.87 mg alpha-HCH/kg (on a fat basis).

In a number of countries, important food items have been analysed for the presence of alpha-HCH. The levels, mainly in fat-containing food products, ranged up to 0.05 mg/kg product, except in milk and milk products (up to 0.22 mg/kg) and in fish and processed meat products (up to 0.5 mg/kg on a fat basis). A slow decrease over the years has been noted.

Food is the main source for general population exposure to alpha-HCH. In total-diet studies in the Netherlands and the United Kingdom, mean concentrations of 0.01 and 0.002-0.003 mg/kg food, respectively, were found. The United Kingdom data indicate a downward trend since 1967. In the USA, the average daily intake of alpha-HCH was 0.009-0.025 µg/kg body weight during the period 1977-1979, and 0.003-0.016 µg/kg body weight during the period 1982-1984.

In a few countries, the concentration of alpha-HCH has been determined in human blood, serum, or plasma. The mean (in some cases median) concentration was < 0.1 µg per litre (ranging from undetectable levels to 0.6 µg per litre). In one country, however, a mean concentration of 3.5 (range 0.1-15.0) µg/litre was reported. Alpha-HCH was detected in approximately one third of the blood samples.

The concentrations in human adipose tissue and breast milk are reported to be low (respectively < 0.01-0.1 and < 0.001-0.04 mg/kg on a fat basis). Total-diet studies have shown daily intake levels of the order of 0.01 µg/kg body weight per day or lower. These concentrations are decreasing slowly over the years.

Alpha-HCH appears to be a universal environmental contaminant. Concentrations are only decreasing slowly, in spite of measures taken to prevent its spread into the environment.

1.4 Kinetics and metabolism

In rats, alpha-HCH is rapidly and almost completely absorbed from the gastrointestinal tract. After intraperitoneal injection, approximately 40-80% of the alpha-HCH was excreted via the urine and 5-20% via the faeces. In rats, the highest concentrations have been found in liver, kidneys, body fat, brain and muscles, and substantial deposition occurs in fatty tissue. The alpha-HCH concentrations in the liver of sucklings were twice as high as those observed in the liver of the mothers. In rats, the brain to blood and depot fat to blood ratios were 120:1 and 397:1, respectively.

The biotransformation of alpha-HCH in rats involves dechlorination. The major urinary metabolite is 2,4,6-trichlorophenol; other identified metabolites include 1,2,4-, 2,3,4-, and 2,4,5-trichlorophenol and 2,3,4,5- and 2,3,4,6-tetrachlorophenol. 1,3,4,5,6-Pentachlorocyclohex-1-ene has been found in rat kidneys and also in *in vitro* studies on chicken liver. A glutathione conjugate is formed in the liver.

The half-life for clearance from the fat depot is 6.9 days in female rats and 1.6 days in males.

1.5 Effects on organisms in the environment

Alpha-HCH has low toxicity for algae, 2 mg/litre generally being the no-observed-effect level.

Summary and Evaluation

In a long-term study, *Daphnia magna* showed a no-observed-effect level of 0.05 mg/litre. Alpha-HCH is moderately toxic for invertebrates and fish. The acute $L(E)C_{50}$ values for these organisms are in the order of 1 mg/litre. In short-term studies with guppies and *Oryzia latipes*, 0.8 mg/litre was without effect.

In three-month studies with *Salmo gairdneri* at dose levels of 10-1250 mg/kg diet, there were no effects on mortality, behaviour, growth, or enzyme activities in liver and brain.

Short- and long-term studies with a snail *(Lymnea stagnalis)* showed an EC_{50} (based on mortality and immobilization) of 1200 µg/litre. Inhibition of egg production occurred at a concentration of 250 µg/litre. A 50% reduction in the overall reproductivity was found at 65 µg/litre.

No data are available on effects on populations and ecosystems.

1.6 Effects on experimental animals and *in vitro* test systems

The acute oral LD_{50} values for mice lie between 1000-4000 and for rats between 500-4670 mg/kg body weight. The poisoning signs are mainly those of stimulation of the central nervous system.

A 90-day study with rats showed growth depression at a concentration of 250 mg/kg diet. Histological and enzyme level changes in the liver indicated enzyme induction at 50 mg/kg or more. At these dose levels there were also indications of immunosuppression. Liver weights were already increased at 10 mg/kg diet (equivalent to 0.5 mg/kg body weight). The no-observed-adverse-effect level in this study appeared to be 2 mg/kg diet (equivalent to 0.1 mg/kg body weight per day).

No adequate long-term toxicity studies or reproduction and teratogenicity studies have been reported.

Studies with various strains of *Salmonella typhimurium* yielded no evidence of mutagenicity either with or without metabolic activation. Tests with *Saccharomyces cerevisiae* were also negative, but a test for unscheduled DNA synthesis in rat hepatocytes *in vitro* gave an equivocal result.

Studies to determine carcinogenic potential have been carried out with mice and rats at dose levels from 100 to 600 mg/kg diet. Hyperplastic nodules and/or hepatocellular adenomas were found in studies on mice. In one study the dose levels exceeded the maximum tolerated dose. Two mice studies and one rat study, using dose levels of up to 160 mg/kg diet in mice and 640 mg/kg diet in rats, did not show any increase in the incidence of tumours.

The results of the studies on initiation-promotion and mode of action and the mutagenicity studies indicate that the alpha-HCH-induced tumorigenicity observed in mice has a non-genetic mechanism.

Alpha-HCH has been shown to cause a clear increase in the activity of liver enzymes even at 5 mg/kg diet (equivalent to 0.25 mg/kg body weight). A dose of 2 mg/kg body weight did not affect aminopyrine demethylation or the DNA content of the liver.

1.7 Effects on humans

When workers at a lindane-producing factory, with a geometric mean exposure of 7.2 years (1-30), were investigated, it was concluded that occupational HCH exposure did not induce signs of neurological impairment or perturbation of "neuromuscular function".

2. IDENTITY, PHYSICAL AND CHEMICAL PROPERTIES, ANALYTICAL METHODS

2.1 Identity of primary constituent

Common name   Alpha-hexachlorocyclohexane (alpha-HCH)

Chemical formula $C_6H_6Cl_6$

Chemical structure (see Appendix 1)   Alpha-HCH is a stereoisomer of gamma-HCH, the active ingredient of lindane (> 99% gamma-HCH). It differs in the spatial orientation of the hydrogen and chlorine atoms on the carbon atoms:

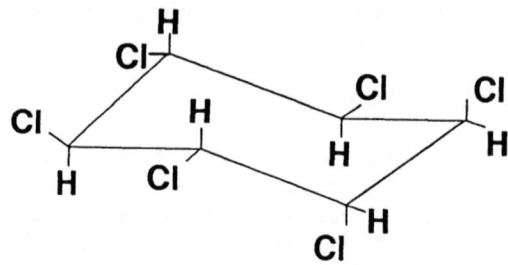

Relative molecular mass   290.9

CAS chemical name   1α,2α,3β,4α,5β,6β-hexachlorocyclohexane

Common synonyms   Alpha-benzenehexachloride (alpha-BHC)

CAS registry number   319-84-6

RTECS registry number   GV3500000

2.2 Physical and chemical properties

Some physical and chemical properties are summarized in Table 1.

Table 1. Some physical and chemical properties of alpha-hexachlorocyclohexane

Melting point	158 °C
Boiling point	288 °C
Vapour pressure (20 °C)	2.67 Pa (0.02 mmHg)
Relative density (20 °C)	1.87 g/cm^3
Solubility water (28 °C) organic solvents (20 °C)	2 mg/litre acetone 139 g/litre chloroform 63 g/litre ethanol 18 g/litre petroleum ether 7-13 g/litre xylene 85 g/litre
Stability	considerable stability in acids, unstable in alkaline conditions
n-Octanol/water partition coefficient (log P_{ow})	3.82

2.3 Analytical methods

Hildebrandt et al. (1986) and Wittlinger & Ballschmiter (1987) described in detail the appropriate analytical methods, i.e. air sampling by adsorption, extraction, purification, and determination using high resolution gas chromatography. Sampling was conducted by pumping air first through a glass fiber filter and then a layer of silica gel. An internal standard was used. The extraction was carried out with dichloromethane, and the extract was evaporated. Preseparation was on silica gel and elution with a mixture of hexane and dichloromethane. For the determination, use was made of high resolution capillary gas chromatography with electron capture detection and a mass selective detector.

Eder et al. (1987) described in detail three different analytical methods for the determination of HCHs in sediments. Sediments are extracted with a solvent or mixture of solvents and are concentrated or fractionated. The alpha-HCH is determined by gas chromatography with electron capture detection or other methods.

3. SOURCES OF HUMAN AND ENVIRONMENTAL EXPOSURE

Alpha-HCH does not occur naturally. It is released to the environment as a result of the use of technical-grade HCH and the inappropriate disposal of the residue resulting from the purification of lindane.

Alpha-HCH is basically a by-product (and impurity) in the manufacturing of lindane (> 99% gamma-HCH). Technical-grade HCH, which is synthesized from benzene and chlorine in the presence of ultraviolet light, consists of:

65-70%	alpha-HCH
7-10%	beta-HCH
14-15%	gamma-HCH (lindane)
≈ 7%	delta-HCH
≈ 1-2%	epsilon-HCH
≈ 1-2%	other components

Purification of lindane produces a residue, consisting almost entirely of non-insecticidal HCH isomers (mainly alpha- and beta-), which can be used as an intermediate for the production of trichlorobenzene and other chemicals.

Alpha- and beta-HCH have been used in mixtures with gamma-HCH (as "HCH" or "fortified HCH") in agriculture and in wood protection.

4. ENVIRONMENTAL TRANSPORT, DISTRIBUTION, AND TRANSFORMATION

4.1 Transport and distribution between media

MacRae et al. (1967) studied the persistence and biodegradability of alpha-HCH in two clay soils. The rate of treatment was 15 mg/kg soil, and incubation periods of 0, 15, 30, 50, 70, and 90 days were used. Only very small amounts of alpha-HCH could be detected in non-sterilized soils after 70 days, indicating a low level of persistence and biodegradation. However, the losses were much slower in sterilized soils, and were probably due to volatilization.

Tsukano (1973) studied the factors affecting the disappearance of alpha-HCH from rice field soil after granular application (0.05 mg/litre) to the surface water. The surface water and soil were analysed at intervals, and alpha-HCH was found to disappear rapidly with a half-life of about 5 days. Following translocation of alpha-HCH (1 mg/litre) onto flooded levelled soil, a decrease in the level in water and steady increase in the level in soil occurred. After 7 days the concentration in soil reached a maximum. Data from a soil column study showed that alpha-HCH moved downwards with the percolating water.

Suzuki et al. (1975) studied the persistence of alpha-HCH in three different types of soil. The persistence was found to be determined by environmental factors such as the action of microorganisms, co-distillation, evaporation from soil, and the contents of water and organic matter in the soil.

In a study by Wahid & Sethunathan (1979), the sorption and desorption of alpha-HCH by 12 soils from rice-growing areas in India were studied using ^{14}C label. The soils showed striking differences in their ability to adsorb alpha-HCH, the sorption values ranging from 40 to 95% of total added alpha-HCH. After oxidation of the soil with hydrogen peroxide, the sorption was lower (5-46%). Organic matter was the most important factor governing the sorption and desorption, but pH, exchange acidity, exchangeable sodium and magnesium, and electrical conductivity also affected the results.

Korte (1980) summarized the behaviour of alpha-HCH in the environment, especially in soil and plants.

4.2 Biotransformation

4.2.1 Biodegradation

Heritage & MacRae (1977, 1979) investigated the degradation of alpha-HCH (final concentration 5 mg/litre) by a washed suspension of *Clostridium sphenoides* in the absence of oxygen at 30 °C. The alpha-isomer was no longer detectable after 4 h. Apparently the degradation proceeded via delta-3,4,5,6-tetrachlorocyclohexene (delta-TCCH). Aerobically grown facultative anaerobes actively dechlorinated ^{36}Cl-alpha-HCH during anaerobic incubation with glucose, pyruvate or formate as substrates, but this dechlorination was slower than in the case of lindane.

When incubation studies were performed under anaerobic or aerobic conditions, the dechlorination of ^{36}Cl-labelled alpha-HCH by mixed soil flora and by pure cultures of *Citrobacter freundii, C. butyricum,* and *C. pasteurianum* was 6.5%, 13.9%, 97.4%, and 53.2%, respectively, within 6 days of incubation. Again, alpha-HCH degraded more slowly than lindane (Jagnow et al., 1977).

Screening experiments to study the possible isomerization of lindane to alpha-HCH, using *C. freundii, Serratia marcescens, Pseudomonas putida,* and other bacterial species, gave negative results (Haider, 1979).

Doelman et al. (1985) carried out laboratory studies on the degradation of alpha-HCH, at a concentration of approximately 5300 mg/kg, in a polluted Dutch sandy loam soil with 6.5% organic matter. They found during 20 weeks constant degradation rates of 10 mg/kg per day under anaerobic conditions and 14 mg/kg per day under aerobic conditions. At a lower concentration (approximately 3900 mg/kg) the average degradation rate appeared to be higher (24 mg/kg per day) under both aerobic and anaerobic conditions. The degradation was ascribed to microbial processes.

Studies in 1986 on HCH-polluted soil (personal communication by P. Doelman and A. Zehnder to the IPCS) indicate that alpha-HCH degrades considerably better in aerobic conditions (aerated slurry) than in anaerobic conditions (non-aerated slurry) both in the laboratory and in soil in greenhouses (Slooff & Matthijsen, 1988). Assuming the degradation process to be a first-order reaction, MacRae et al. (1984) calculated from laboratory studies (soil with 4.0% organic carbon) half-lives of 125 and 48 days under aerobic and anaerobic conditions, respectively.

In a study by Doelman et al. (1988a), microbial soil sanitation was applied to calcareous alkaline sandy loam soil that was polluted with a mixture of HCH isomers. Under anaerobic conditions, microbial degradation in the Dutch climate (soil temperature of 5-17 °C) did not occur, and even the low concentration of the easily degradable gamma-HCH did not decrease.

Microbial soil sanitation of alpha-HCH-polluted calcareous sandy loam soil systems has been investigated. The soil systems involved were aerated moist soil and continuously aerated and intermittently aerated soil slurries. Degradation of alpha-HCH appeared to proceed according to a first-order reaction. It was fastest during the first 4 weeks, even though soil temperatures were lowest during this period. The percentage degradation during the first 4 weeks was 40, 80, and 37%, respectively, for the three soil systems. The degradation rate gradually decreased with time even if the temperature increased. Addition of microbial biomass did not significantly affect the alpha-HCH degradation. In a continuously aerated thick slurry system, the alpha-HCH concentration was reduced from approximately 420 to 15 mg/kg. Thus, alpha-HCH degradation will occur in regions with a temperate climate, provided that the soil is aerobic (Doelman et al., 1988b).

A field investigation into the distribution of HCHs was carried out by Chessells et al. (1988) using soil from an agricultural area treated with BHC-20 (HCH composition: 70% alpha-HCH, 6.5% beta-HCH, 13.5% gamma-HCH, and 5% delta-HCH. Although the concentration of alpha-HCH was the highest of the HCHs, the alpha-isomer disappeared more rapidly than beta-HCH. Furthermore, soil organic carbon content was found to be of primary importance. A significant decrease in isomer concentration was observed when soil moisture content was high and was attributed to microbial degradation favoured by these conditions.

4.2.2 Abiotic degradation

Alpha-HCH is broken down by ultraviolet light but at a slower rate than lindane. Ultraviolet irradiation, using a 15-watt low pressure mercury lamp, of alpha-HCH in 2-propanol solution for 10 h resulted in the production of an isomer of pentachlorocyclohexene. This substance may be produced by hydrogen abstraction of the radiation-induced pentachlorocyclohexyl radicals (Hamada et al., 1982).

4.2.3 Bioaccumulation/Biomagnification

4.2.3.1 Algae

A study was carried out to determine the bioconcentration of alpha-HCH by an alga *(Cladophora)* during a period of 48 h. At concentrations of alpha-HCH in water of 4.4 and 31 µg/litre, the bioconcentration factors were 341 and 180, respectively (Bauer, 1972).

In a study by Canton et al. (1975), *Chlorella pyrenoidosa* cells taken from a log-phase culture were exposed for 96 h to alpha-HCH (> 95%) concentrations of 10, 50 or 800 µg/litre, and after 15, 30, and 180 min the cells were analysed. At all dosage levels the average bioconcentration from water was about 200-fold (153-267). There seemed to be a tendency for alpha-HCH to accumulate in the cytoplasm rather than the cell wall. When the cells were subsequently placed in clean water, the elimination was rapid (15 min).

When Canton et al. (1977) investigated the accumulation and elimination of alpha-HCH (> 95%) in marine algae *(Chlamydomonas* and *Dunaliella)* in studies lasting a few days, both processes were found to take place rapidly, (i.e. in less than 30 min). The average concentration factor was 2700 in *Chlamydomonas* and 1500 in *Dunaliella* (on a dry weight basis) and was 12 000 and 13 000, respectively, on a lipid basis. The accumulated alpha-HCH was found primarily in the lipophyllic parts of the cells.

4.2.3.2 Invertebrates

In a study by Canton et al. (1978), *Artemia* was exposed to alpha-HCH (> 95%) levels of 0.01, 0.05 or 0.25 mg/litre and sampled after 0.5, 3, 24, 48, 72, and 96 h. Once equilibrium was reached, the animals were transferred to alpha-HCH-free water and were sampled after 0, 3, 24, 48, 96, and 144 h. The bioconcentration factor was about 60-90 (8000-11 000 on a lipid basis), and equilibrium was reached within 24 h. The elimination half-life was 48-72 h.

Ernst (1979) measured alpha-HCH bioconcentration factors in two marine invertebrates, the mussel *(Mytilus edulis)* and the polychaete *(Lanice conchilega)*, of 105 and 2750, respectively, at 10 °C and an alpha-HCH concentration of 2-5 µg/litre. Species differences and the lipid content of the animals appeared clearly to affect the bioconcentration factor, whereas the effect of temperature seemed to be minimal.

In a study by Yamato et al. (1983), the short-necked clam *(Venerupis japonica)* rapidly absorbed alpha-HCH and the concentration reached a plateau on the third day. The bioconcentration factor was 161 at an alpha-HCH concentration of 1 µg/litre water. The alpha-HCH concentrations on day 6 in organs and tissues were 0.060 and 0.029 mg/kg, respectively. After a 3-day elimination period, the levels were 0.033 and 0.024 mg/kg, respectively.

Mouvet et al. (1985) investigated the presence of alpha-HCH in the aquatic moss *Cinclidotus danubicus* to examine the potential use of this species as an indicator of chlorinated pollutants in fresh water. The moss was sampled 0, 13, 24, and 51 days after having been transplanted in a polluted river, and levels of 0.20-1.33 µg per litre water were found 4 km downstream of an area of industrial discharge. The levels of alpha-HCH in the moss were < 0.025, 0.04-0.57, 0.08-2.37, and 0.81 mg/kg dry weight, respectively, at the time intervals indicated above.

4.2.3.3 Fish

Canton et al. (1975) studied the accumulation and elimination of alpha-HCH by *Chlorella, Daphnia,* and

Poecilia reticulata, and in *Chlorella-Daphnia* and *Daphnia-Poecilia reticulata* systems. In this food-chain study, the following concentration ratios were measured:

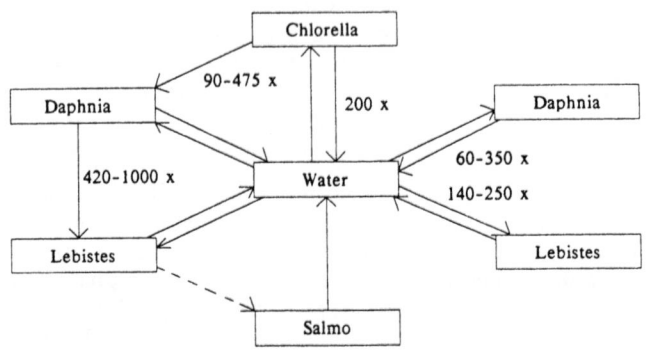

The direct uptake of alpha-HCH from contaminated water appeared to be much greater than the uptake from contaminated food.

In a study with *Salmo gairdneri*, pellets containing alpha-HCH (> 95%) levels of 0, 10, 50, 250, or 1250 mg/kg were fed to the fish, and organs and tissues were analysed after 2, 4, 8, and 12 weeks. There was a dose-related increase in the concentration of alpha-HCH in the organs and tissues. After about 4-8 weeks (depending on the type of tissue and dose level) a maximum concentration was reached, which then slowly decreased. This suggests that after a few weeks a balance is reached between the accumulation process (absorption of alpha-HCH by the intestinal wall) and the elimination process (via the gills and faeces). There is probably also a dilution effect resulting from growth and biotransformation (Canton et al., 1975).

Ernst (1977) concluded from kinetic studies that biomagnification of alpha-HCH does not occur. Compared with bioaccumulation from water alone, the entry of alpha-HCH into the food chain *Chlorella* -> *Daphnia* -> *Poecilia* (guppy) caused only a slight increase in biomagnification in daphnids (factor 1.5), although in the case of the guppies a greater increase in concentration ratio (3-4) was noted.

In a study by Canton et al. (1978), guppies (3-4 weeks old) were exposed to alpha-HCH (> 95%) concentrations of 0.01, 0.05, or 0.14 mg/litre. When after 0.5, 3, 24, 48, 72, 96, and 120 h the animals were analysed, the average concentration factor was about 500 for all alpha-HCH concentrations (about 17 000 on a lipid basis). Equilibrium was reached within 24 h for the lower concentrations and within 48 h at the highest concentrations. The elimination was rapid, the initial concentration being halved in 10 h.

Sugiura et al. (1979) studied bioaccumulation in the carp *(Cyprinus carpio)*, brown trout *(Salmo trutta fario)*, golden orfe *(Leuciscus idus melanotus)*, and guppy *(Poecilia reticulata)*. Alpha-HCH was dissolved in water to a concentration of 1 mg/litre under steady-state conditions (time period not specified), and the equilibrium bioconcentration factors for the four types of fish were 330, 605, 1216, and 588, respectively.

Based on the data given in section 5.1.5.2 concerning the concentration of alpha-HCH in the muscle and fat of bream collected in the River Elbe, the bioconcentration factor is between 10 000 and 50 000 (Arbeitsgemeinschaft für die Reinhaltung der Elbe, 1982).

In a study by Yamato et al. (1983), guppies *(Poecilia reticulata)* rapidly bioaccumulated HCH isomers and the tissue concentration reached a plateau on the fourth day (the alpha-HCH concentration in the water was 1 μg per litre). The bioconcentration factor (concentration in fish/concentration in water) was 706. The concentration in the guppies decreased on the first day after the fish were transferred to HCH-free water.

4.2.3.4 Bioconcentration in humans

Geyer et al. (1986) found that in industrialized countries more than 90% of the exposure to HCHs derives from food. The mean concentration of alpha-HCH in human adipose tissue (on a fat basis) was found to be 0.03 mg/kg in the Federal Republic of Germany and 0.02 mg/kg in the Netherlands. The mean bioconcentration factor (on a lipid basis), calculated on the basis of the concentration in the diet (1.3 and 0.3 µg/kg, respectively) and levels in adipose tissue, was 20.0 ± 8 (range 11.5-32.5).

4.3 Isomerization

Deo et al. (1981) studied the isomerization of alpha-HCH in sterile aqueous solution over a period of 4 weeks and found a slow conversion of alpha-HCH to other HCH isomers.

5. ENVIRONMENTAL LEVELS AND HUMAN EXPOSURE

5.1 Environmental levels

5.1.1 Air

Tanabe et al. (1982) found alpha-HCH in 24 samples of air over the Western Pacific, Eastern Indian, and Antarctic Oceans at an average concentration of 0.29 ng/m^3 (0.022-1.4 ng/m^3).

In a study by Strachan et al. (1980), samples of atmospheric precipitation in the form of snow (1976; 17 samples) and rain (1976 and 1977; 81 samples) collected around the Canadian side of the Great Lakes, as well as inland, were analysed. Alpha-HCH was found in the snow samples as a trace (1 ng/litre) and in the rain samples at levels of 1-40 ng/litre.

Air samples were taken near a road with heavy traffic, as well as in a suburban residential area, near Ulm, in Germany. The alpha-HCH levels were 0.22-1.3 ng/m^3 in the location with heavy traffic and 0.11-1.1 ng/m^3 in the rural area. It was concluded that the concentrations in the lower troposphere under various meteorological conditions reflect regional input and long-range transport (Wittlinger & Ballschmiter, 1987).

In 1972, alpha-HCH air concentrations of 0.28 ng per m^3 in non-polluted areas of Germany, and 2.15 ng/m^3 in the polluted Ruhr area were determined (Hildebrandt et al., 1986).

The average concentration of alpha-HCH in 55 air samples collected in Delft, the Netherlands, in 1979-1980 was 0.25 ng/m^3 (maximum concentration: 1.2 ng/m^3) (Slooff & Matthijsen, 1988).

5.1.2 Water

5.1.2.1 Rain water

Rain water sampled in 1983 in Bilt, the Netherlands, contained an average alpha-HCH concentration of 0.01 (< 0.01-0.02) μg/litre (Slooff & Matthijsen, 1988).

5.1.2.2 Fresh water

During the period 1969-1977, 1826 water samples were taken at 99 sampling sites in the Netherlands. The highest concentrations of alpha-HCH were found in the River Rhine and its tributaries. The concentrations varied between 0.01-0.3 µg/litre during the period 1969-1974, but in 1974 there was a sudden decrease and the subsequent concentrations were all below 0.1 µg/litre. A sampling trip by boat made along the River Rhine from Rheinfelden in Switzerland to Rotterdam in the Netherlands proved that the source of alpha-, beta-, and gamma-HCH was located in the upper Rhine. In the River Meuse, the levels were all below 0.1 µg/litre during the period 1969-1977 (Wegman & Greve, 1980).

Since 1969, alpha-, beta-, and gamma-HCH concentrations have been measured regularly in the Rivers Rhine, Meuse, and West-Scheldt and in other surface waters in the Netherlands. Alpha-HCH levels have been below 0.05 µg per litre in the River Rhine since 1974/1975, and were of the order of 0.02 µg/litre or less in the West-Scheldt during the period 1973-1985. In the River Meuse, the concentration of alpha-HCH was between 0.01-0.02 µg/litre. In other areas, for instance agricultural and greenhouse horticulture areas, the levels of the individual HCHs ranged from 0.01-1.0 µg/litre with incidental higher peaks (up to 0.5 µg/litre) probably resulting from the use of lindane (Slooff & Matthijsen, 1988).

Concentrations of HCH isomers in solution and in suspension (particle-bound) in the Meuse and Rhine estuary were determined in 1974. The average concentrations of dissolved and suspended alpha-HCH were 20 and 0-6 ng per litre, respectively. In 1981, the concentration of dissolved alpha-HCH in coastal waters of the Netherlands was 0.9-1.6 ng/litre, whereas that of suspended alpha-HCH (only one measurement) was 5.3 ng/litre (Slooff & Matthijsen, 1988).

In 1970-1971, the levels of alpha-HCH were 0.66-1.5 µg/litre in the surface water of the River Elbe near Hamburg, Germany, and 0.155-2.4 µg/litre in the River Rhine near Karlsruhe. However, a significant decrease was observed in the mid-1970s. In 1974, 2.7 µg per litre was found in the upper Rhine, but by 1976-1977 the levels had decreased to 1-9 ng/litre (Hildebrandt et al., 1986).

The Arbeitsgemeinschaft der Elbe (the Elbe Study Group) investigated the presence of alpha-HCH in the River Elbe from Schnackenburg to the North Sea in 1981-1982 and found a mean concentration of 0.023 (< 0.001-0.15) µg per litre. During the period February to November 1988, the alpha-HCH concentration was 0.001-0.022 µg/litre (Arbeitsgemeinschaft der Elbe, 1988).

When certain rivers in Yorkshire, England, were analysed for alpha-HCH in 1966, the concentration varied from 0.001 to 0.43 µg/litre. In 1968, the highest value was 0.543 µg/litre, and the water from six other rivers contained an average of 0.001-0.004 µg/litre (highest level: 0.34 µg/litre) (Lowden et al., 1969).

In Japan, 60 water samples were examined in 1974 and 0.1 µg alpha-HCH/litre was detected in three of the samples (personal communications by A. Hamada and by T. Onishi to the IPCS, July 1989).

5.1.2.3 Sea water

Atlas & Gias (1981); Bidleman & Leonard (1982); Oehme & Stray (1982); and Oehme & Mano (1984) analysed sea water from areas such as the North Pacific, Arabic Sea, Persian Gulf, Red Sea, Lillestrum, Bear Island, and Spitsbergen. The alpha-HCH concentrations varied from 0.03 to 1.8 ng per litre (Slooff & Matthijsen, 1988).

In June-July 1986, the alpha-HCH in the surface water (5 m) of the North Sea ranged from 1-2 ng/litre (Umweltbundesamt, 1989).

5.1.3 Soil/Sediment

Herrmann et al. (1984) studied the presence of alpha-HCH in sediment along the Husum estuary and in the adjacent North Frisian Wadden Sea. The mean concentrations varied in the different sampling stations from 0.33 to 1.40 µg/kg sediment, while the concentrations in bladder wrack *(Fucus vesiculosus)* varied from 0.7-1.2 µg/kg.

Edelman (1984) analysed 96 samples of the upper 10 cm of the soil from 38 natural reserves in the Netherlands for alpha-HCH and gamma-HCH. In 94 of the samples alpha-HCH was detected at levels below 1 µg/kg (Slooff & Matthijsen, 1988).

When sediment from eight different rivers, harbours, and sites close to dumping areas in the Netherlands were analysed for the presence of alpha-, beta-, and gamma-HCH, the median alpha-HCH levels were between 4 and 213 µg per kg dry matter (Slooff & Matthijsen, 1988).

In 1974, 60 sediment samples were analysed in Japan and 10 µg alpha-HCH/kg was detected in five of the samples (personal communications by A. Hamada and by T. Onishi to the IPCS, July 1989).

5.1.3.1 Dumping grounds

In the Netherlands, soil has been polluted with HCHs at various locations as a result of their manufacture during the 1950s (spillage during production, storage, and handling), and concentrations up to a few grams of HCHs/kg dry soil have been found. Further pollution has been caused by the dumping of chemical waste and its use in the levelling of certain areas. From these dumping areas dispersal of the chemical waste can occur by leaching or wind erosion from open storage depots. In certain polluted areas, high concentrations of HCHs, mainly alpha- and beta-HCH, have been found more than 2 m below ground level. In 18 locations in the Netherlands, the average concentration of alpha-HCH in sewage sludge in 1981 was between 5 and 70 µg/kg dry matter. Pollution of ground water was also detected, but this was restricted to the vicinity of the production areas. Horizontal transportation of HCHs in ground water appeared to be limited (Slooff & Matthijsen, 1988).

5.1.4 Food and feed

The presence of alpha-HCH in a number of important food items has been determined in France by Laugel (1981). In milk and milk products (2688 samples) the average level was 0.05 mg/kg (ranging from undetectable to 0.22 mg/kg), in meat (37 samples) it was 0.01 mg/kg (ranging from undetectable to 0.02 mg/kg), and in animal fat (67 samples) it was 0.02 mg/kg product (ranging from undetectable to

0.06 mg/kg. In other food items alpha-HCH was not detectable (< 0.005 mg/kg).

Table 2 gives the mean alpha-HCH levels in a large number of samples of various food items from the Federal Republic of Germany reported by Hildebrandt et al. (1986).

Table 2. Alpha-hexachlorocyclohexane concentrations (mg/kg) in various food items[a]

Food items	1973-78	1979-83	1973-83
Meat[b]			0.003-0.02
Meat products[b]		0.007-0.037 (0.26)[e]	
Animal fat[b]			0.003-0.008 (0.09)[e]
Game[b]			0.019-0.367
Poultry[b]	0.003-0.004	0.003-0.016 (0.17)[e]	
Chicken eggs			< 0.001-0.003
Fish		0.002-0.011	
Milk and milk products[b]	0.015[e]	0.01-0.03	
Cow's milk[b,c]		0.004	
Butter[b,d]		0.02-0.03	
Vegetable oil and margarine[b]	0.01		
Oil seeds, nuts, pulses		0.001-0.042	
Fruit, vegetables, potatoes			< 0.0001
Cereals			0.0002-0.007
Cereal products			up to 0.14

[a] From: Hildebrandt et al. (1986).
[b] Determinations made on a fat basis
[c] WHO (1986).
[d] Anon (1984).
[e] Maximum value

In six samples of cows milk collected from six locations in Switzerland, the levels of alpha-HCH were 9.5-27 mg/kg on a fat basis (Rappe et al., 1987).

Skaftason & Johannesson (1979) analysed 35 samples of butter from Iceland during 1968-1970 and found a level of mean alpha-HCH of 87 ± 38 µg/kg. In 1974-1978, 32 samples were studied and all contained alpha-HCH, the mean concentration being 58 ± 21 µg/kg.

In a total-diet study in the United Kingdom, 24 samples of each food group were analysed for alpha-HCH. The following concentrations (mean and range) were found: bread, not detected (nd); other cereal products, < 0.0005 (nd-0.002); carcass meat, < 0.0005 (nd-0.006); offal, < 0.0005 (nd-0.007); meat products, eggs, green vegetables, potatoes, fresh fruit, nd; poultry, 0.003 (nd-0.025); fish, 0.0005 (nd-0.008); oil and fats, 0.0005 (nd-0.003); milk, 0.0005 (nd-0.002); dairy products, 0.006 (nd-0.02) mg/kg product. Imported meat products were also analysed during the period 1981-1983, and concentrations of up to 0.5 mg/kg were measured. Imported retail cereal products collected in 1982 contained alpha-HCH levels of up to 0.03 mg/kg and animal feed stuffs collected in 1984 had levels of up to 0.02 mg/kg (HMSO, 1986).

Various types of pulses were analysed during the period 1986-1987, and 31 out of 142 samples contained alpha-HCH residues at levels of up to 0.03 mg/kg. Processed pork and poultry, sampled during the period 1985-1987, contained alpha-HCH at levels of up to 3.2 (mean 0.2) and 0.1-2.0 (mean 0.8) mg/kg product, respectively (26 out of the 86 samples were positive). Of other processed meat products, 631 samples were negative. Retail milk and dairy products were analysed during the period 1984-1987, and 499 of the 849 samples contained alpha-HCH residues at a mean concentration of 0.01-0.03 mg/kg (highest level, 0.06 mg/kg). Samples of eel muscle (1124 eels from 62 sites) were analysed during the period 1986-1987, and mean concentrations were 0.001-0.03 mg/kg (highest level, 0.4 mg/kg). Peanut butter and vegetable oils were analysed during the period 1985-1987, and 95 samples showed mean concentrations of < 0.01-0.03 mg/kg product (16 of the samples were positive) (HMSO, 1989).

The mean residue level of alpha-HCH in milk samples collected during spring 1983 from 359 bulk transporters representing 16 counties, municipalities, and districts of Ontario was 5.3 µg/kg butter fat. Alpha-HCH was found in over 90% of the samples (Frank et al., 1985).

5.1.5 Terrestrial and aquatic organisms

5.1.5.1 Plants

Samples of three types of mosses and four types of lichens (in total 13 samples) were collected in the Antarctic Peninsula (Graham Land) in 1985, and alpha-HCH was detected in most of them at a mean concentration of 0.4 (0.20-1.15) µg/kg (Bacci et al., 1986).

In a study by Gaggi et al. (1986), fallen leaves (at the end of their natural life-cycle) and lichens were collected in 1984 at sites near Florence and Siena, Italy, in a woodland hilly area away from primary pollution sources. The leaves were from ten different species of trees and two different lichen species were involved. The average levels of alpha-HCH in leaves and lichen were 37 (16-61) µg/kg dry weight and 27 (25-29) µg/kg dry weight, respectively. The same authors reported that the levels of alpha-HCH in various plant species collected in 14 countries were 0.5-2140 µg/kg dry weight.

5.1.5.2 Fish and mussels

Martin & Hartman (1985) analysed 60 fish samples from nine locations in the north-central part of the USA and found concentrations of 5-27 µg alpha-HCH/kg (wet weight) in 36% of the samples. The frequency with which alpha-HCH was detected in fish from the different rivers varied between 17 and 100%.

In a study by Saiki & Schmitt (1986), samples of three to five adult bluegills *(Lepomis macrochirus)* and common carp *(Cyprinus carpio)* were collected at eight sites in three rivers in California, USA, in 1981. Alpha-HCH concentrations in carp of up to 0.036 mg/kg on fat basis were reported, but the concentrations in bluegill were lower.

Cowan (1981) studied the extent of pollution of Scottish coastal waters by HCHs using *Mytilus edulis* as biological indicator. The levels of alpha-HCH at the 118 sites sampled ranged from < 6 to 23 µg/kg dry weight.

Environmental Levels and Human Exposure

The fish and shellfish sampling programme carried out by the United Kingdom Ministry of Agriculture, Fisheries, and Food between 1977-1984 was directed mainly to areas around the coasts of England and Wales. The levels of alpha-HCH, which varied between the different fish and shellfish species and also between the collection sites, ranged from < 0.001 (nd) to 0.06 mg/kg wet weight. The concentration in fish muscle was < 0.001 mg/kg wet weight (Franklin, 1987).

The mean alpha-HCH concentration in the muscle of flounders collected off the North Sea coast of Germany in 1986 was 2.5 µg/kg (nd-5.0 µg/kg) (Umweltbundesamt, 1989). Bream collected from different locations in the River Elbe (between Schnackenburg and the North Sea) contained 0.007-0.066 mg alpha-HCH/kg in muscle tissue and 0.9-2.2 mg/kg in adipose tissue (Arbeitsgemeinschaft für die Reinhaltung der Elbe, 1982), while the same species collected from 15 rivers and lakes in the Federal Republic of Germany contained (on a fat basis) up to 468 µg per kg (Umweltbundesamt, 1989).

Freshwater fish from different rivers in the Federal Republic of Germany were analysed during the period 1973-1981, and in the first 3-4 years the alpha-HCH levels were mainly between 0.01 and 0.02 mg/kg fresh weight. However, a clear decrease then took place and most of the samples were below 0.01 mg/kg fresh weight, with the exception of certain types of fish such as the eel and fish from industrially contaminated areas (Hildebrandt et al., 1986).

In 1981-1983, shellfish and molluscs collected in the Federal Republic of Germany contained < 0.001-0.20 mg alpha-HCH/kg fresh weight. Eels collected in the North Sea and Baltic Sea contained alpha-HCH levels of 0.011 mg per kg and 0.033 mg/kg fresh weight, respectively. Flounders and herrings caught in the North Sea contained 0.002 and 0.008 mg/kg fresh weight, respectively, but in the Baltic Sea the levels were about twice as high (Hildebrandt et al., 1986).

5.1.5.3 *Birds*

An average alpha-HCH residue level of 0.05 mg/kg was found in 17 adult herons in 1964 (HMSO, 1969).

In a study by Sierra & Santiago (1987), alpha-HCH concentrations were determined in 23 barn owls *(Tyto alba Scop.)* from Leon, Spain. The mean levels (and range) in muscle, liver, fat, brain, and kidneys (in total 91 samples) were 0.242 (0.019-0.591), 0.323 (0.009-0.830), 1.073 (0.691-1.499), 0.238 (0.007-0.676), and 0.710 (0.051-2.381) mg/kg (wet weight), respectively.

Faladysz & Szefer (1982) analysed adipose fat from seven species of diving ducks at their winter quarters in the Southern Baltic. Residues of alpha-HCH were found in all of the 37 specimens of long-tailed duck at mean concentrations (on a fat basis) of 3.4 (0.17-18) and 1.5 (0.23-6) mg/kg for female and male ducks, respectively.

5.1.5.4 *Mammals*

Skaftason & Johannesson (1979) analysed 24 samples of the fat of reindeer living in an area of the eastern and south-eastern parts of Iceland where the use of pesticides is negligible. Alpha-HCH was found in all samples at a mean level of 70 ± 22 µg/kg. These results are in agreement with those of Benson et al. (1973), who found an average of 77.5 µg/kg in the subcutaneous fat of wild Idaho moose living in a forest area where pesticides were used very restrictively. Skaftason & Johannesson (1979) analysed samples of body fat from 10-year-old sheep in 1974 and found an average of 51 ± 12 µg/kg.

Norström et al. (1988) investigated the contamination by organochlorine compounds of Canadian arctic and subarctic marine ecosystems by analysing the adipose tissue and liver of polar bears *(Ursus maritimus;* 6-20 animals per area) collected from 12 areas between 1982 and 1984. There was a difference in tissue distribution; liver contained only alpha-HCH, but 29% of the HCH in adipose tissue was beta-HCH. Adipose tissue contained 0.3-0.87 mg alpha-HCH per kg on a fat basis.

The mean concentrations of alpha-HCH in the kidney fat of roe (86 samples) collected in five areas of Germany in 1985-1986 were about 7-12 µg/kg fat, the maximum value being about 50 µg/kg fat (Umweltbundesamt, 1989).

5.2 General population exposure

From the data presented in section 5.1 it is evident that food is the main source of exposure of the general population to alpha-HCH.

5.2.1 Total-diet studies

In a total-diet study carried out in the United Kingdom during 1966-1985, food purchased in 21 towns throughout the country was prepared by cooking. The study covered 20 to 24 food groups, and the number of total-diet samples examined varied from 22 to 25 samples. The calculated mean alpha-HCH residue levels in the total diet for the periods 1966-1967, 1970-1971, 1974-1975, 1975-1977, 1979-1980, 1981, and 1984-1985 were 0.003, 0.002, 0.002, 0.0015, 0.001, < 0.0005, and < 0.0005 mg/kg, respectively (Egan & Hubbard, 1975; HMSO, 1982, 1986, 1989).

Gartrell et al. (1985a) conducted a study to determine the dietary intake of pesticides in the USA in 1978-1979. The samples, purchased from retail outlets, were representative of the diets of adults in 20 cities, and consisted of about 120 individual food items. The daily intake of alpha-HCH in 1977, 1978, and 1979 was 0.011, 0.009, and 0.010 µg/kg body weight, respectively. In a similar way, samples were collected in 10 cities in 1978-1979 consisting of about 50 items of infant food and 110 items of toddler food. The daily intake of alpha-HCH in 1977, 1978, and 1979 was, respectively, 0.031, 0.034, 0.033 µg/kg for infants and 0.025, 0.029, and 0.029 µg/kg body weight for toddlers, respectively (Gartrell et al., 1985b).

Total-diet studies conducted in the USA by the FDA before 1982 were based on a "composite sample approach" regardless of the diet involved. Later on they were based on dietary survey information and allowed the "total diet" of the population to be represented by a relatively small number of food items for a greater number of age-sex groups. The daily intakes of alpha-HCH during 1982-1984 for the age groups 6-11 months, 2 years, 14-16-year-old females, 14-16-year-old males, 25-30-year-old females, 25-30-year-old males, 60-65-year-old females, and 60-65-year-old males were 7.2, 16.1, 6.1, 7.3, 4.5, 5.9, 3.3, and 3.7 ng/kg body weight, respectively (Gunderson, 1988).

In a total-diet study in the Netherlands in 1977, the average concentration of alpha-HCH in 100 samples was 0.01 mg/kg on a fat basis. The highest level was 0.05 mg/kg (Greve & van Hulst, 1977).

5.2.2 Air

Guicherit & Schulting (1985) measured the atmospheric concentration of alpha-HCH in the Netherlands and calculated an average daily intake by inhalation for a 70-kg person of 5 ng. The equivalent value for the Federal Republic of Germany was calculated to be 32 ng, which is about 1% of the total daily intake via the various routes (Hildebrandt et al., 1986).

5.2.3 Concentrations in human samples

Alpha-HCH concentrations in human samples are a good indication of the total exposure of the general population.

5.2.3.1 Blood

Blood samples of Dutch citizens analysed in 1978, 1980, 1981, and 1982 (70, 48, 127, and 54 samples, respectively), contained less than 0.1 µg alpha-HCH/litre (Greve & Wegman, 1985). Blok et al. (1984) analysed the blood of 65 healthy volunteers in the Netherlands (34 female and 31 male) and detected alpha-HCH in less than one third of the samples. The median concentration for both groups was below the detection limit (0.1 µg per litre), but levels of up to 0.4 µg/litre were measured.

Polishuk et al. (1970) studied the presence of alpha-HCH in the blood of 24 pregnant women and 23 infants living in Israel. The mean concentration was 0.6 ± 0.3 µg per litre in the women and 0.5 ± 0.3 µg/litre in the infants.

In 1975, Reiner et al. (1977) analysed the serum and plasma of 82 women and 65 men (with an average age of 42) living in a town in Yugoslavia. In 57 of the 147 samples, alpha-HCH was found at a mean concentration of 3.3 ± 0.5 µg/litre (range, 0.1-15.0 µg/litre). Similar values were found in other parts of the country in 1976-1979 (Krauthacker et al., 1980).

The median concentration of alpha-HCH in whole blood of 118 people in the Federal Republic of Germany was reported to be 0.98 µg/litre (range, nd-2.06) (Bertram et al., 1980).

5.2.3.2 *Adipose tissue*

The alpha-HCH concentrations of 567 samples of adipose tissues of Dutch citizens analysed during 1968-1983 varied from < 0.01 to 0.1 mg/kg (on a fat basis). The highest levels occurred during the period 1968-1976 (Greve & van Harten, 1983; Greve & Wegman, 1985).

In a study by Niessen et al. (1984), specimens of subcutaneous adipose tissue from 48 infants (34 under the age of 1 year, 14 in their second year of life) were examined during 1982-1983 in the Federal Republic of Germany. The average concentration of alpha-HCH was 0.01 mg/kg fat (range, nd-0.02 mg/kg). The average concentration was highest (0.02 mg/kg fat) for the age-range 0-6 weeks. Bertram et al. (1980) found a median concentration of 0.03 mg/kg fat (range, nd-0.35) in 72 samples of adipose tissue from people in the Federal Republic of Germany. Hildebrandt et al. (1986) summarized the results of nine studies carried out in the Federal Republic of Germany during 1969-1983. The mean alpha-HCH concentrations (568 samples) ranged from 0.01 to 0.03 mg/kg fat.

Mes et al. (1982) analysed 99 samples of adipose tissue from autopsies of accident victims from different areas of Canada. Nearly all the samples (97%) contained alpha-HCH, the average concentration of which was 0.004 mg/kg wet weight (range, 0.001-0.043 mg/kg).

In 1974, 360 samples of adipose tissue were collected in eight regions of Japan and the mean level of alpha-HCH was 0.031 mg/kg tissue (Takabatake, 1978).

Twenty-nine samples of adipose tissue were taken at necropsy and 24 at surgery in the Poznan district of Poland and compared with 100 samples from residents of the

Warsaw area. In Poznan the mean concentration of alpha-HCH was 0.013 ± 0.033 mg/kg, while in Warsaw it was 0.008 ± 0.001 mg/kg (Szymczynski et al., 1986).

5.2.3.3 *Breast milk*

Breast milk is a major route for the elimination of organochlorine pesticides in women. In a Swedish study, the levels of alpha-HCH in breast milk were found to be related to the dietary habit. Levels in lacto-vegetarians were lower than those in women eating a mixed diet, and these were lower than those found in mothers using a mixed diet that regularly included fatty fish from the Baltic (Noren, 1983).

In a study by Fooken & Butte (1987), the variation of residue levels in breast milk during lactation was investigated in five women (aged 23-36) in the Federal Republic of Germany. Alpha-HCH concentrations of up to 0.009 mg/kg fat were measured, and no essential changes in residue level occurred over the lactation period.

Residues of alpha-HCH in breast milk during the periods, 1974-1975 and 1979-1980 in the Federal Republic of Germany were reported to be 0.03 and 0.02 mg/kg milk on a fat basis, respectively (Anon., 1984).

In the Federal Republic of Germany, more than 7100 samples of breast milk were analysed from 1969-1984. These studies were carried out by 20 authors, and the results were summarized by Hildebrandt et al. (1986). The mean concentrations of alpha-HCH ranged from 0.01-0.04 mg/kg on a fat basis. In one case a mean concentration of 0.21 mg/kg was found in 320 samples. During the period investigated, a slow decrease in the mean concentration of alpha-HCH was observed. The average concentration in breast milk in the same country (2709 samples) in 1979-1981 was 0.024 mg/kg on a fat basis (Fooken & Butte, 1987). In 1981-1983, 132 samples of breast milk were analysed and the average level was 0.001 mg alpha-HCH/kg milk fat (Cetinkaya et al., 1984).

Tuinstra (1971) analysed 36 individual samples of breast milk, collected in 1969, from young mothers (18-32 years of age) living in the Netherlands. A median alpha-HCH concentration of 0.01 mg/kg milk (on a fat basis) was found (range, nd-0.04). When 278 samples of breast milk, collected in 11 maternity centres in the Netherlands, were analysed for the presence of alpha-HCH, the median alpha-HCH concentration was < 0.01 mg/kg (on a fat basis) (Greve & Wegman, 1985).

Vukavic et al. (1986) measured the alpha-HCH concentration in 59 samples of colostrum collected during autumn 1982 (26 samples) and spring 1983 (33 samples) in Yugoslavia from healthy nursing mothers on the third day after delivery. The alpha-HCH levels were significantly lower in the autumn than in the spring (mean concentrations of 0.49 ± 0.09 and 1.50 ± 0.26 µg/litre whole colostrum, respectively).

Mes et al. (1986) studied 210 breast milk samples from five different regions of Canada and measured a mean alpha-HCH concentration of 7 µg/kg (on a fat basis). Davies & Mes (1987) studied 18 breast milk samples from Canadian, Indian, and Inuit mothers in Canada, whose fish consumption was comparable to the national level. The level of alpha-HCH in milk fat of the indigenous population was 5 µg/kg, which was the same value as that obtained from a national survey.

6. KINETICS AND METABOLISM

6.1 Absorption and elimination

The intestinal absorption rate for alpha-HCH was 97.4% after the administration of an HCH mixture to male rats (Albro & Thomas, 1974).

The total excretion in rats after a single intraperitoneal (ip) ^{36}Cl-labelled alpha-HCH dose of 200 mg/kg body weight was 80% of the dose in the urine and 20% in the faeces (Koransky et al., 1963; Koransky et al., 1964; Noack et al., 1975). In a study in rats with ^{36}Cl-labelled alpha-HCH, a low excretion rate was found. ^{36}Cl was detected in the excreta up to 40 days after a single ip dose (Koransky et al., 1963). During continued dosing alpha-HCH was observed to stimulate its own degradation (Noack et al., 1975). The decrease in rat liver alpha-HCH levels after an initial increase, observed by Eichler et al. (1983), was assumed to be due to this effect.

When ^{14}C-labelled alpha-HCH was administered intraperitoneally to male mice (ddY-strain, 4 weeks old) at a dose level of 22 µg, the average percentage of urinary excretion of radioactivity in 3 days was 37% (Kurihara & Nakajima, 1974).

6.2 Distribution

One day after an ip injection of a mixture of ^{14}C- and ^{36}Cl-labelled alpha-HCH into rats (200 mg/kg body weight in rapeseed oil), the highest level of radioactivity was found in fat, skin, and bones plus muscles (18.2, 13.1, and 11.9%, respectively, after 4 days). Much lower levels were found in other organs or tissues (up to 1% in liver and kidneys and 0.28% in the central nervous system. In the faeces and urine, 3.9 and 7.9%, respectively, were found after 4 days (Koransky et al., 1963). In other studies with rats, higher concentrations were found in liver, kidneys, body fat, brain, and muscle (Portig & Vohland, 1983; Kuiper et al., 1985). In a 90-day study in rats, marked deposition of alpha-HCH was found in renal fat; the concentrations exceeded those obtained in a similar study on beta-HCH (Greve & van Hulst, 1980; Kuiper

Kinetics and Metabolism

et al., 1985). In lactating rats given a single oral dose 5 days after birth, the alpha-HCH concentrations in the livers of the sucklings were twice as high as those observed in the livers of the mothers (Wittich & Schulte-Hermann, 1977).

Vohland et al. (1981) studied the distribution of alpha-HCH in the brain and depot fat of rats after the administration of 200 mg/kg body weight by gavage. With an average blood concentration of 1.5 µg/litre, the brain to blood, and depot fat to blood ratios were 120:1 and 397:1, respectively, whereas with a blood concentration of 17.7 mg/litre the ratios were 5:1 and 82:1, respectively.

Nagasaki (1973) orally administered alpha-HCH to male mice at concentrations of 100, 250 or 500 mg/kg for 24 weeks, and found high residual levels of this isomer in liver and adipose tissue. Similarly, Macholz et al. (1986) reported that a 30-day administration of alpha-HCH to rats resulted in high residues of this isomer in fat, kidneys, and adrenal tissue.

In the brain, alpha-HCH is stored preferentially in the white matter (Stein et al., 1980; Portig et al., 1989).

6.3 Metabolic transformation

6.3.1 Rat

When Sprague-Dawley weanling female rats were administered 2 mg alpha-HCH/rat per day in peanut oil for 7 days, the alpha-HCH was metabolized to 2,4,6- and 2,4,5-trichlorophenol, with an excretion ratio of 2,4,6- to 2,4,5-trichlorophenol of 1.3:1. This study also indicated that pre-treatment with alpha-HCH alters the metabolism of lindane in rats (Freal & Chadwick, 1973).

The biotransformation of alpha-HCH in rats involves dechlorination (Kraus, 1975). The dose-dependent decrease in liver glutathione concentrations indicates the formation of a glutathione conjugate in this organ (Noack & Portig, 1973; Portig et al., 1973; Kraus, 1975). Such a decrease does not occur in the brain or kidneys (Noack & Portig, 1973).

The major urinary metabolite in rats is 2,4,6-trichlorophenol, a compound reported by IARC (1987) to be carcinogenic for animals (Portig et al., 1973; Stein & Portig, 1976; Stein et al., 1977). Other metabolites that have been identified are 1,2,4-trichlorophenol, 2,3,4-trichlorophenol, 2,4,5-trichlorophenol, 2,3,4,5-tetrachlorophenol, and 2,3,4,6-tetrachlorophenol (Noack et al., 1975; Stein et al., 1977; Macholz et al., 1982). In addition, chlorothiophenols (not specified) have been detected, and 1,3,4,5,6-pentachlorocyclohex-1-ene has been identified in the kidneys of rats (Macholz et al., 1983).

Artigas et al. (1988) have identified several lindane metabolites (tetra-, penta-, and hexachlorocyclohexenes, and tetra- and pentachlorobenzenes) in rat brain homogenates by gas chromatography-mass spectrometry. Male Wistar rats were orally administered 30 mg alpha-HCH/kg and were sacrificed 5 h later. The cerebella of the animals were analysed and the following metabolites were found: 3.6/4.5-PCCH, 3.5/4.6-PCCH, HCCH, pentachlorobenzene, and HCB. HCCH was the major metabolite (about 100 μg per kg) while levels of the other metabolites were mainly below 5 μg/kg. Alpha-HCH was present at 17.2 mg/kg tissue. This study showed that the HCH isomers are cleared from the brain via different metabolic pathways.

Isomerization of alpha-HCH to lindane did not occur after repeated dosage (Eichler et al., 1983).

6.3.2 Bird

In a model 4-week feeding study on poultry using four HCH isomers, the rate of degradation of the individual HCH isomers in broilers followed the order: delta > gamma > alpha > beta. Biotransformation (to one or more of the other HCH isomers) was not detected (Szokolay et al., 1977b).

In a study by Foster & Saha (1978) on the *in vitro* metabolism of alpha-HCH in chicken livers, the first metabolite was identified as an isomer of pentachlorocyclohexane.

6.3.3 Human

When Engst et al. (1978) analysed the urine of occupationally exposed workers (apparently to technical-grade

HCH in manufacturing processes), they found, apart from alpha-, beta-, gamma-, and delta-HCH, traces of hexa- and pentachlorobenzene, gamma- and delta-pentachlorocyclohexane, pentachlorophenol, 2,3,4,5-, 2,3,4,6-, and 2,3,5,6-tetrachlorophenol, and several trichlorophenols, as well as the glucuronides of several of these metabolites. The pentachlorocyclohexenes, tetrachlorophenol, hexachlorobenzene, and pentachlorophenol were also identified in the blood.

6.4 Retention and biological half-life

The half-life for the clearance of alpha-HCH from depot fat was found to be 6.9 days in female rats and 1.6 days in male rats (Stein et al., 1980; Portig, 1983).

Vohland et al. (1981) and Portig & Vohland (1983) studied the kinetics of alpha-HCH in Wistar rats, and observed that, after a single oral dose of 200 mg/kg body weight, the approximate half-life in females for the elimination from brain was 6 days.

The retention of alpha-HCH in rat brain after a single dose is greater than that of beta- and gamma-HCH (Stein et al., 1980).

7. EFFECTS ON LABORATORY MAMMALS AND IN VITRO TEST SYSTEMS

7.1 Single exposure

7.1.1 Acute toxicity

In mice oral LD_{50} values have been found to range from 1000 to 4000 mg/kg body weight, depending on the vehicule, while in rats values of 500-4674 mg/kg body weight have been obtained. Riemschneider (1949) determined a LD_{50} (oral intubation in olive oil) for rats of 1500 mg/kg body weight. The signs of poisoning were those of nervous system stimulation: excitation, hunched posture, rough fur, dyspnoea, anorexia, tremors, convulsions, and cramps (Hoffmann, 1983; WHO, 1986).

7.2 Short-term exposure

7.2.1 Oral

In a 90-day study on rats carried out with dose levels of 0, 2, 10, 50, or 250 mg alpha-HCH/kg diet, reductions in white blood cell count were noted in several groups of animals. Growth was decreased at 250 mg/kg diet, and at this dose level the number of erythrocytes and protein excretion in the urine were elevated in female animals. At levels of 50 and 250 mg/kg, the activities of liver aminopyrine-N-demethylase and aniline hydroxylase were increased while those of blood aspartate aminotransferase (ASAT) and creatine phosphokinase were decreased. Liver weights were increased at dose levels of 10, 50, and 250 mg/kg. Enlargement of liver parenchyma cells (with a foamy/hyaline appearance of the cytoplasm) and accentuation of the plasmalemma, indicative of proliferation of smooth endoplasmatic reticulum (SER), occurred at levels of 50 and 250 mg/kg. At the 250-mg/kg level, there were increases in the relative weights of heart, kidneys, and adrenals. In addition, serum levels of immunoglobulins G and M showed a decrease at 50 and 250 mg/kg diet (Kuiper et al., 1985).

Macholz et al. (1986) reported that the administration of 1000 mg alpha-HCH/kg to rats for 30 days resulted in growth retardation and liver mass increase. High residue levels of alpha-HCH were identified in fat, kidneys, and adrenal tissue.

7.2.2 Other routes

7.2.2.1 Intravenous

In a study by van Asperen (1954), groups of 12-15 male and female albino mice (8-10 weeks of age) were given an intravenous injection of alpha-HCH (in peanut oil). The dose levels were 480 or 960 μg/mouse (equivalent to approximately 32 and 64 mg/kg body weight, respectively). No deaths occurred within 7 days.

7.2.2.2 Subcutaneous

Groups of 13-21 male and female albino mice (8-10 weeks of age) were given a subcutaneous injection of alpha-HCH at dose levels ranging from 3 to 20 mg/animal (equivalent to approximately 200 to 1330 mg/kg body weight, respectively). With doses of up to 4 mg, no death occurred within 7 days, but with 4.5 mg, 8 mg, and 20 mg, 8, 25, and 90%, respectively, of the animals died (van Asperen, 1954).

7.3 Skin and eye irritation; sensitization

No data on skin and eye irritation or sensitization have been reported.

7.4 Long-term exposure

7.4.1 Rat oral study

When groups of 10 female and 10 male weanling Wistar rats were administered diets containing 0, 10, 50, 100, or 800 mg alpha-HCH/kg diet (in corn oil) for 107 weeks, the highest dose level resulted in growth retardation, increased mortality, and slight kidney damage. With dose levels of 100 or 800 mg/kg, liver enlargement and histopathological changes in the liver were found. However, there were no liver changes at 50 mg/kg diet (Fitzhugh et al., 1950).

7.5 Reproduction, embyrotoxicity, and teratogenicity

No information on reproduction, embryotoxicity, or teratogenicity is available.

7.6 Mutagenicity and related end-points

Alpha-HCH did not induce mutations in *Salmonella typhimurium* test strains TA98, TA100, TA1535 or TA1537 either with or without rat liver metabolic activation (Lawlor & Haworth, 1979). A test for point mutations in *Saccharomyces cerevisiae* XV 185 14 C was also negative (Shahin & von Borstel, 1977). In addition, the compound produced no mutations in *Allium cepa* roots (Nybom & Knutsson, 1947). A test for unscheduled DNA synthesis in rat hepatocytes *in vitro* produced an equivocal result (Althaus et al., 1982).

A mutagen test strain of *Bacillus subtilis* (TKJ5211) showed a higher sensitivity for his[+] reversion than the parental strain HA101 when treated with UV and UV-mimetic chemicals. However, a negative result was obtained when alpha-HCH dissolved in DMSO was used at a dose level of 5 mg/ml (Tanooka, 1977).

A DNA repair test was carried out with stationary-phase cultures of *B. subtilis* HLL3g and HJ-15 strains in which the size of growth inhibition zones of repair-proficient and repair-deficient cells for vegetative cells and spores was determined. There was no effect at a dose level of 5 mg alpha-HCH (in benzene) per ml (Tanooka, 1977).

The available data are inadequate to make an assessment of the mutagenic potential.

7.7 Carcinogenicity

Appraisal

The reported studies on the carcinogen effects of alpha-HCH on mice and rats have some short-comings. In most cases, very high dose levels were tested. Nevertheless, it is clear from the results that alpha-HCH, at high dose levels, produces nodular hyperplasia and hepatocellular carcinomas in mice (the incidence varying according to the strain) and also in rats (low incidence), but only at higher dose levels.

The results of the studies on initiation-promotion and mode of action indicate that the neoplastic response observed with alpha-HCH is most likely due to a non-genotoxic mechanism.

7.7.1 Mouse

When 20 male ICR/JCL mice (aged 5 weeks) were administered a diet containing 600 mg alpha-HCH/kg diet for 26 weeks, increased liver weight was observed. In all treated mice there were liver tumours, which were characterized histologically as benign tumours and malignant tumours with atypical liver cells. Unfortunately, insufficient details were reported (Goto et al., 1972a,b).

In a study by Hanada et al. (1973), 6-week-old DD mice (10-11 of each sex per group) were given diets containing 0, 100, 300, or 600 mg alpha-HCH/kg diet for 32 weeks, followed by a control diet for 5-6 weeks. The control group consisted of 20 female and 21 male animals. During the experiment several animals died. The numbers of hepatomas in the four groups surviving for 36-38 weeks were 0/29 (control), 1/16 (100 mg/kg), 9/10 (300 mg/kg), and 13/15 (600 mg/kg). Alpha-fetoprotein was not detected in the serum of animals with hepatomas.

When 8-week-old male DD mice, divided into groups of 20 or 38 animals, were fed a diet containing 0, 100, 250, or 500 mg alpha-HCH/kg for 24 weeks, the two highest dose levels induced an increase in liver weight. At the four respective dose levels, the incidence of nodules classified as nodular hyperplasia was 0/20, 0/20, 30/38 (79%), and 20/20 (100%) and that of hepatocellular carcinoma was 0/20, 0/20, 10/38 (26%), and 17/20 (85%) (Ito et al., 1973b).

Following the oral administration of 100, 250 or 500 mg alpha-HCH/kg to male DD mice for 24 weeks, hepatocellular tumours were found in all mice treated with 500 mg/kg and in 17 of the 20 mice that received 250 mg/kg (Nagasaki, 1973).

Nagasaki et al. (1975) studied the tumorigenic effects of a diet containing 0 or 500 mg alpha-HCH/kg, fed for

24 weeks to groups of male and female DDY, ICR, DBA/2, C57BL/6, and C3H/He mice (13-29 of each sex per group), male Wistar rats, and male golden Syrian hamsters. It was found that alpha-HCH induced liver tumours in male and female mice but not in rats and hamsters. The histological changes in the liver of mice were much greater than those induced in rats and hamsters. Male animals were more susceptible to the tumorigenic action (i.e. liver nodules) than females. Among the different strains of mice, a difference in susceptibility was observed. The occurrence of liver nodules varied from 16.7 to 100% and the incidence of hepatocellular carcinomas varied from none to 65%. The DDY mouse strain was the most sensitive and the C57BL/6 the least sensitive strain.

Ito et al. (1976) studied the reversibility of liver tumours induced by alpha-HCH (99.0%). Male 8-week-old DDY mice were fed a diet containing 0 or 500 mg/kg for 16, 20, 24, and 35 weeks and then fed a basal diet without alpha-HCH for 4, 8, and 12, or 4, 8, 12, 16, 24, and 36 weeks. In total 341 mice were used, of which 21 were fed the compound for 16 weeks. A total of 300 mice were fed the diet with alpha-HCH for 20 or more weeks and 20 control mice were fed the basal diet for 72 weeks. At the various intervals indicated, 12-20 mice were killed. The incidence of liver tumours increased progressively during continuous administration of alpha-HCH, but when its administration was discontinued some tumours disappeared. After 24 weeks of administration most tumours were nodular hyperplasias with only a few well-differentiated hepatocellular carcinomas. However, 60 or 72 weeks after the beginning of the study most of the liver tumours were hepatocellular carcinomas. The findings suggested that nodular hyperplasia was usually reversible.

Two groups of male HPBC57B1 black mice (6-9 weeks old) were fed a diet containing 500 mg/kg alpha-HCH (99.8%) per diet, 48 mice being used as controls and 75 mice being administered alpha-HCH. From each group, 4-9 mice were killed at 1, 3, 4, 8, 14, 21, 30, 33, 44, and 50 weeks after the initiation of treatment. Progressive liver enlargement was first noticed at 3 weeks, hepatic nodules at 21 weeks, and emaciation at 30 weeks. Histopathological liver alterations included hypertrophy of centrolobular hepatocytes first seen at 1 week and the merging of adjacent megalocytic zones at 3 weeks. At 21 weeks, adenomas were seen in two out of seven mice, at 30 weeks in seven out of eight mice, and at 33, 44, and 50 weeks in all the mice studied. Under the condition of this study, neither hepatocellular carcinomas nor metastases in the lungs were detected (Tryphonas & Iverson, 1983).

7.7.2 Rat

When groups of 10 male and 10 female weanling Wistar rats were fed throughout their life on diets containing 10, 50, 100, or 800 mg alpha-HCH (> 98% pure) per kg, no increase in tumour incidence was found. However, only a limited number of organs were examined microscopically (Fitzhugh et al., 1950).

In a study by Ito et al. (1975), male Wistar rats (5-8-weeks old) were divided into seven groups and administered alpha-HCH diets containing 0, 500 (two groups), 1000 (three groups), or 1500 mg α-HCH/kg diet. The duration of the treatment for the different groups was 72 weeks for the controls, 24 or 48 weeks at 500 mg/kg, 24, 48, or 72 weeks at 1000 mg/kg, and 72 weeks at 1500 mg/kg. In the liver, oval cells and bile duct cell proliferation were found in the groups fed 1000 or 1500 mg/kg after 48 and 72 weeks. Cell hypertrophy was found in all the groups, the increase in severity depending on the dose level and the duration of administration. In the two groups fed 500 mg/kg and the group fed 1000 mg/kg for 24 weeks no nodular hyperplasia or hepatocellular carcinomas were found. Nodular hyperplasia developed in the groups fed 1000 mg/kg (48 and 72 weeks) or 1500 mg/kg (72 weeks) in 42, 76, and 77% of the animals, respectively. Hepatocellular carcinomas were found only in the groups fed 1000 or 1500 mg/kg for 72 weeks (1/16 and 3/13 animals, respectively).

In a series of studies, an oral dose of 20 mg/kg body weight was administered daily to female rats during periods of 4.5, 13.5, or 23.5 months. Liver enzyme induction was found at all intervals, white foci and nodules were present after 13.5 months, and one animal had a hepatocellular carcinoma after 23.5 months (Schulte-Hermann & Parzefall, 1981). The value of this study was reduced by the very low number of animals (4-6 per group) used at each interval.

7.7.3 Initiation-promotion

In a study on 8-week-old white male mice (25-30 per group) of strain DD, the influence of alpha-HCH on tumour induction by polychlorinated biphenyls (PCBs) was tested and vice versa. Whereas 500 mg PCB/kg diet induced nodular hyperplasia and hepatocellular carcinomas in the liver of male mice after 32 weeks, exposure to alpha-HCH at dose levels of 50, 100, or 250 mg/kg diet, only resulted in both type of tumours at the highest dose level. The incidence of nodular hyperplasia was 23/30 (77%) and that of hepatocellular carcinoma was 8/30 (27%). However, 50 or 100 mg alpha-HCH/kg diet, in combination with 250 mg PCB per kg diet (PCB alone did not induce tumours), induced nodular hyperplasia (approximately 30%) and hepatocellular carcinoma (approximately 5%). It seems that PCBs promote the induction of liver tumours by alpha-HCH (Ito et al., 1973a).

In studies on rats, alpha-HCH showed a tumour-promoting action towards the hepatocarcinogenic effects of aflatoxin B1, diethylnitrosamine, and nitrosomorpholine (Schulte-Hermann & Parzefall, 1981; Schulte-Hermann et al., 1981; Angsubhakorn et al., 1981). In one test, alpha-HCH produced only a slight liver tumour-promoting effect in rats after initiation with N-nitrosodiethylamine (Ito et al., 1983). However, in another study on the same species the compound had an inhibitory effect on the hepatocarcinogenic action of 3-methyl-4-dimethylaminoazobenzene and DL-ethionine (Thamavit et al., 1974).

Nagasaki et al. (1975) studied the influence of 3-methylcholanthrene, 1-naphthyl isothiocyanate, and p-hydroxypropiophenone on the induction of liver tumours by alpha-HCH. Eight groups of 24 mice received a diet containing either 500 mg alpha-HCH/kg diet in combination with 67 mg methylcholanthrene/kg, 600 mg 1-naphthyl isothiocyanate/kg or 1000 mg p-hydroxypropiophenone/kg or just one of the four compounds. A control group with the basal diet was also used. The induction of mouse liver tumours by alpha-HCH was not inhibited by the concomitant feeding of 1-naphthyl isothiocyanate or p-hydroxypropiophenone. However, 3-methylcholanthrene slightly inhibited their induction by alpha-HCH.

In a study by Schröter et al. (1987), the tumour-initiating activity of alpha-HCH was studied by examining for phenotypically altered foci in female Wistar rats. Groups of three to eight rats were used and, after removing the median and right liver lobes, 200 mg alpha-HCH/kg body weight was administered followed by phenobarbital at 50 mg/kg body weight per day for 15 weeks. Liver foci were identified by means of the gamma-glutamyltransferase (GGT) reaction and by morphological alterations. No evidence of initiating activity was found. In another part of the study, the promoting activity was investigated. A single dose of N-nitrosomorpholine (250 mg/kg body weight by gavage) was followed by the administration of 0.1, 0.5, 2.0, 7.0, or 20.0 mg alpha-HCH/kg body weight per day for 4, 15, and 20 weeks. The criteria used were growth and phenotypic changes of foci as end-points. It was concluded from the study that alpha-HCH is a tumour promotor. Both the number and size of altered foci were enhanced by alpha-HCH doses of 2 mg/kg or more. The tumour-promoting action was generally associated with liver enlargement and induction of monooxygenases or other specific enzymes.

Schulte-Hermann et al. (1983) carried out three experiments with Han-Wistar rats using, in experiment 1, 39 female rats (8-24 months old) and, in experiments 2 and 3, 41 male (2 years old) rats. Alpha-HCH (200 mg/kg in corn oil) was administered orally as a single dose, while the control group received only corn oil. Beginning 25 h after the dosing, ^{3}H-thymidine was injected intravenously five times at intervals of 6 h (experiment 2) or 8 h (experiment 3), and the animals were killed 18 (experiment 2) or 3 h (experiment 3) after the last dose of ^{3}H-thymidine. The effect of age on the incidence of spontaneous foci was studied in experiment 1. Foci of putative preneoplastic cells were detected in the livers of untreated rats of both sexes, especially at 1 and 2 years of age. These foci exhibited markers similar to those of their counterparts in carcinogen-treated rats, such as cytoplasmic basophilia, clearness of cytoplasm, or expression of gamma-glutamyl transferase. Rates of DNA synthesis in foci were higher than in normal liver cells and were increased by single doses of liver mitogens assumed to promote liver tumour development. Thus cells in the spontaneous foci appeared to possess a defect in the growth control, rendering them more susceptible to endogenous and exogenous growth stimuli.

The incorporation of orally administered radiolabelled thymidine into liver DNA was determined in SIV-50-SD rats 24 h after a single oral gavage dose of 2.9, 29.1, 58.2, or 291 mg alpha-HCH/kg. Alpha-HCH was found to stimulate liver DNA synthesis at 58.2 mg/kg (Büsser & Lutz, 1987).

7.7.4 Mode of action

Sagelsdorff et al. (1983) studied the relevance to the carcinogenic action of alpha-HCH of covalent binding to mouse liver DNA. Three strains of mice were used (NMRI, CF_1, and $C6B3F_1$), and alpha-HCH was administered by oral gavage and ^{14}C-thymidine by the intraperitoneal route. In all three strains, a similar low covalent binding index or DNA damage/dose (values ranging from 0.17-0.28) was found. There was no quantitative correlation with the carcinogenicity potency of alpha-HCH.

Iverson et al. (1984) studied the ability of alpha-HCH to bind to macromolecules from male HPB black mouse liver. *In vivo* and *in vitro* binding studies with ^{14}C-alpha-HCH and hepatic microsomes from untreated and phenobarbital-pretreated mice showed no preferential binding of alpha-HCH to protein or DNA. The results suggest that the neoplastic response observed with alpha-HCH results from a non-genotoxic mechanism.

7.8 Special studies

7.8.1 Effect on liver enzymes

After a single oral administration to female rats of 5 mg alpha-HCH/kg body weight or more the rate of aminopyrine demethylation and the liver DNA content were both increased, but at 2 mg/kg body weight these effects did not occur (Schulte-Hermann et al., 1974). In a further study, the liver cytochrome P450 concentration in male rats after a single oral administration was elevated at all tested dose levels, 25 mg/kg body weight being the lowest (Seifart & Buchar, 1978). After alpha-HCH was given to male rats at dose levels of 5, 10, 20, 50, or 200 mg/kg feed for 2 weeks, aniline hydroxylase and aminopyrine demethylase activities were increased at all dose levels (den Tonkelaar et al., 1981).

7.8.2 Neurotoxicity

Appraisal

Alpha-HCH has been shown to have no effect on motor nerve conduction velocity or the fronto-occipital EEG in rats fed 1000 mg alpha-HCH/kg diet for 30 days. This isomer is a mild antagonist of pentylenetetrazol-induced convulsions but increases the tonic/clonic activity and the lethality of picrotoxin when administered intraperitoneally to mice. It decreases the accumulation of cerebellar cyclic GMP and prohibits the increase of cGMP caused by gamma-HCH in mouse brain. Alpha-HCH has been demonstrated to inhibit GABA-mediated chloride ion uptake in mouse brain, and this effect is believed to play a primary role in the CNS action of this isomer.

In a study by Vohland et al. (1981), alpha-HCH did not give rise in brain tissue to appreciable quantities of hydrophobic metabolites such as 2,4,6-trichlorophenol. It had a weak protecting action against convulsions induced by pentylenetetrazole (PTZ). The intensity and duration of the PTZ-antagonistic effects after a single oral dose were related to the alpha-HCH content of the brain.

In a 30-day study on groups of 15 male Wistar rats fed alpha-HCH at levels of up to 1000 mg/kg diet, there was no effect on the fronto-occipital electroencephalogram or on the motor conduction velocity of the tail nerve (Müller et al., 1981).

The effect of alpha-HCH on body temperature, food intake, and body weight was studied in Wistar rats (eight males and eight females) given a single 30-mg/kg oral dose of alpha-HCH in olive oil. Controls received only olive oil. Alpha-HCH treatment induced no significant decrease in core temperature 5 h after treatment, and no decrease in food intake or growth was observed (Camon et al., 1988).

Fishman & Gianutsos (1987) studied the effects of an intraperitoneal injection of alpha-HCH (99.0%) in corn oil (80-480 mg/kg body weight) on the accumulation of cerebellar cyclic GMP in male CD-1 mice. Alpha-HCH decreased the accumulation of cerebellar cyclic GMP and also prevented the increase in cyclic GMP resulting from lindane treatment. Furthermore, alpha-HCH inhibited the binding of ^{3}H-TBOB (a ligand for the GABA-A-receptor-linked chloride channel) in mouse cerebellum.

Fishman & Gianutsos (1988) compared the CNS-related pharmacological and biochemical effects of gamma-HCH and the non-convulsant isomer alpha-HCH. The studies were carried out on male CD-1 mice injected intraperitoneally with a single alpha-HCH (in corn oil) dose of 80-400 mg/kg body weight. Alpha-HCH inhibited the myoclonic jerk and tonic/clonic activity of PTZ but increased the tonic/clonic activity and lethality of picrotoxin (PIC) (PTZ and PIC were given as a single ip injection of 50 mg/kg and 20 mg/kg body weight, respectively). The highest dose of alpha-HCH caused a significant decrease in motor activity. Gamma-HCH inhibited the binding of ^{3}H-TBOB to mouse whole brain membranes. Furthermore, this isomer is a weak inhibitor of GABA-stimulated uptake of ^{36}Cl into mouse brain neurosynaptosome preparations *in vitro*. The non-seizure-inducing alpha-HCH has biochemical and pharmacological effects in the CNS which differ from those of the gamma-HCH.

Matsumoto et al. (1988) provided evidence that all HCH isomers are capable of inhibiting GABA-A-mediated chloride channels in the brain, the relative potency being alpha = gamma > delta > beta. Alpha-HCH was also found to be a potent inhibitor of the batrachotoxin-stimulated action potential flux of sodium ions in N18 neuroblastoma cell cultures (Shain et al., 1987).

8. EFFECTS ON HUMANS

8.1 Acute toxicity - poisoning incidents

Several cases of acute poisoning by technical-grade HCH, resulting either from accidents or occupational exposure, have been described (WHO, 1991). Although alpha-HCH constitutes 65-70% of the technical product, it is likely that the most acutely toxic component, i.e. gamma-HCH, played the major role in these incidents. These cases cannot, therefore, assist in the evaluation of alpha-HCH.

8.2 General population

No specific studies relating to alpha-HCH are available.

A study comparing liver cancer deaths in the USA and the "domestic disappearance" of organochlorine pesticides revealed that in 1962, 18 and 15 years after the introduction of DDT and technical-grade HCH, respectively (when an increase in primary liver cancer due to the organochlorines would be manifest), the number of cases of primary liver cancer as a percentage of the total number of liver cancer deaths began a gradual and steady decline (from 61.3% in 1962 to 56.9% in 1972). The death rate (per 100 000 per year) due to primary liver cancer declined from 3.46 to 3.18 during this period (Deichmann & MacDonald, 1977).

8.3 Occupational exposure

The evaluation of the effects of alpha-HCH on occupationally exposed workers is seriously hampered by the fact that most of the relevant studies concern workers who were exposed during the manufacture and handling of lindane or the handling and spraying of technical-grade HCH among other pesticides, and were thus exposed to all HCH isomers plus impurities and other (process) chemicals. Therefore, it is difficult, if not impossible, to relate the observed effects to individual substances. Consequently these studies have only been described in this monograph where they aid the evaluation.

Behrbohm & Brandt (1959) described 26 cases of allergic and toxic dermatitis that arose during the manufacture of technical-grade HCH. Patch testing with pure alpha-, beta-, gamma-, and delta-HCH yielded negative results, but positive reactions were obtained with the residual fractions.

The level of alpha-HCH in 57 healthy workers (with normal liver function, EMG and EEG) at a lindane-manufacturing plant ranged from 10 to 273 µg/litre, whereas it was below the detection limit in control workers. The concentration in the adipose tissue of eight of the exposed workers ranged from 1 to 15 mg alpha-HCH/kg (in extractable lipids) (Baumann et al., 1980, 1981; Brassow et al., 1981; Tomczak et al., 1981).

The mean serum alpha-HCH level of malaria-control workers that sprayed technical-grade HCH for 16 weeks increased from 10 to 78 µg/litre in previously non-exposed workers and from 18 to 77 µg/litre in those that had been exposed during three previous spraying seasons (Gupta et al., 1982).

Nigam et al. (1986) studied 64 employees from a plant manufacturing HCH who were directly or indirectly associated with the production of this insecticide and thus also exposed to chemicals such as benzene and chlorine. The exposed group was composed of 19 "handlers" (who handled and packed the insecticide), 26 "non-handlers" (plant operators and supervisors exposed indirectly to HCH), and 19 maintenance staff (who visited the plant frequently). The control group consisted of 14 workers who had no occupational contact with the insecticide. The exposure period varied up to 30 years. The mean serum alpha-HCH concentrations in the four groups were 21.1 µg/litre (controls), 21.8 µg/litre (maintenance staff), 41.2 µg per litre (non-handlers), and 100 µg/litre (handlers). Lindane and beta- and delta-HCH were also present. The total HCH concentrations were 51.4, 143.6, 265.6, and 604 µg per litre, respectively. Clinical examination revealed that the majority of the workers from the "handler" and "non-handler" groups exhibited paraesthesia of the face and extremities, headache, and giddiness, and some of them also showed symptoms of malaise, vomiting, tremors, apprehension, confusion, loss of sleep, impaired memory, and loss of libido. The same symptoms were found among the maintenance staff but were less severe and less frequent.

Chattopadhyay et al. (1988) studied 45 male workers exposed to HCH during its manufacture and compared them with 22 matched controls. Exposure was mainly via the skin. Paraesthesia of face and extremities, headache, giddiness, vomiting, apprehension, and loss of sleep, as well as some changes in liver function tests, were reported and were found to be related more to the intensity of exposure (as measured by the HCH levels in blood serum) than to the duration of exposure. The measured exposures to total HCH were 13 to 20 times higher than those in the control groups (no detailed figures were reported). Of the total serum HCH, 60-80% was beta-HCH.

9. EFFECTS ON OTHER ORGANISMS IN THE LABORATORY AND FIELD

9.1 Algae

Palmer & Maloney (1955) used alpha-HCH in a preliminary screening test with two cyanobacterium (blue-green alga), two green alga, and two diatom species. The test concentration was 2 mg/litre of water, and the incubation period was 3-21 days. Alpha-HCH was not toxic at this concentration.

When Canton et al. (1975) exposed *Chlorella pyrenoidosa* to alpha-HCH for 96 h at 28 °C (static system), the EC_{50} (growth inhibition) was > 10 mg/litre (maximum solubility in the medium).

In a study by Krishnakumari (1977), cultures of the green alga *Scenedesmus acutus* of 1, 3, or 5 days of age were tested for sensitivity to alpha-HCH at 28 °C, the growth rate being used as a parameter. Alpha-HCH dissolved in ethanol was added at nominal concentrations of 0.5-100 mg/litre water. The alpha-HCH concentrations that caused a reduction in growth in 1-, 3-, and 5-day-old cultures were 10 (or more), 5, and 0.5 mg/kg, respectively.

When *Chlamydomonas* sp. was exposed at a temperature of 20-25 °C in a static system, the no-observed-effect level (based on the growth in 48 h) was > 1.4 mg/litre. A similar result was obtained with *Dunaliella* sp. at 15 °C and a study duration of 48 and 96 h, the NOEL for growth being 1.4 mg/litre (maximum solubility) (Canton et al., 1978).

9.2 Protozoa

The EC_{50} for *Tetrahymena pyriformis* (3 days in closed system at 27 °C) was reported to be 0.75 mg/litre (Mathur et al., 1984).

9.3 Invertebrates

9.3.1 Acute toxicity

The result of acute or short-term toxicity studies lasting a few days on *Artemia salina*, *Daphnia magna*, and *Lymnaea stagnalis* are summarized in Table 3.

Table 3. Acute or short-term toxicity of alpha-hexachlorocyclohexane for invertebrates

Species	Age	Temperature (°C)	Parameter	Concentration (mg/litre)	References
Artemia salina	3 weeks	24	$LC_{50}^{a,b}$	0.5	Canton et al. (1978)
Daphnia magna	<1 day	20	$LC_{50}^{c,d}$	0.8	Canton et al. (1975)
Lymnaea stagnalis	6 months	22	$EC_{50}^{c,e}$	1.2	Canton & Slooff (1977)

[a] synthetic saltwater
[b] 35 days (but exposure time was 4 days)
[c] 48 h
[d] closed system
[e] growth inhibition/mortality or immobilization

9.3.2 Short- and long-term toxicity

9.3.2.1 Crustaceae

In a study by Canton et al. (1975), *Daphnia magna* was exposed to 0, 10, 50, 200, 1000, or 2000 µg alpha-HCH (> 95%) per litre for 25 days. The daphnids were fed *Chlorella pyrenoidosa*. The sensitivity of daphnids to alpha-HCH markedly increased with exposure time. A concentration of approximately 50 µg/litre or less did not lead to death at any time during the whole life cycle of 2 months. Only with 2000 µg/litre was there an influence on reproduction, the EC_{50} for reproduction inhibition being 100 (54-186) µg/litre. The EC_{50} based on mortality and immobilization was 800 (600-1000) µg/litre (see Table 4).

9.3.2.2 Molluscs

In a short-term (2-day) study, groups of five adult snails *(Lymnaea stagnalis L.)* (6 months of age) were exposed to various dose levels. Based on mortality and immobility, the EC_{50} was estimated to be 1200 (600-2300) µg alpha-HCH (> 95%) per litre (Canton & Slooff, 1977).

In a long-term (70-day) study, groups of 10 snails (5 months of age) were exposed to 20, 100, 300, or 600 µg per litre. The study was divided into a pre-exposure period (14 days) during which all egg capsules and the number of eggs per capsule were counted, an exposure period of 40 days during which four groups of adults and five capsules of each group were exposed to alpha-HCH, and a post-exposure period (16 days) during which snails were placed in water to recover. Based on egg production inhibition, the 40-day EC_{50} was 250 µg/litre. The percentage of fertilized eggs per capsule was not affected, and no morphological abnormalities were noticed during embryonic development. Based on the number of eggs that did not hatch, an EC_{50} of 230 µg/litre was determined. Considering a combination of the inhibition of egg production and the mortality of the young during their development, a 50% reduction of the overall reproductivity was found at 65 µg alpha-HCH/litre. These effects did not disappear during the recovery period of 16 days (Canton & Slooff, 1977) (see Table 4).

Table 4. Long-term toxicity of alpha-hexachlorocyclohexane for invertebrates

Species	Age	Temperature (°C)	Duration (days)	Criteria	Concentration (mg/litre)	References
Daphnia magna	adults	19	21	no mortality; no effects on behaviour, appearance or growth; no influence on reproduction (4 groups of offspring)	0.27[a] 0.09 0.27	Janssen et al. (1987)
Lymnaea stagnalis	eggs and adults	22 22	40 40	EC_{50} (egg production inhibition) hatching, overall productivity	0.25 0.065	Canton & Slooff (1977)

[a] water renewal system

9.4 Fish

9.4.1 Acute toxicity

LC_{50} and EC_{50} (mortality and immobilization) values for fish are summarized in Table 5.

9.4.2 Short- and long-term toxicity

During a 3-month study, rainbow trout *(Salmo gairdneri)* (200-250 g) were fed pellets containing 0, 10, 50, 250, or 1250 mg alpha-HCH (purity > 95%) per kg diet. After 2, 4, 8, and 12 weeks, the fish were examined. Growth, microsomal liver enzymes (aniline hydroxylase and aminopyrine demethylase), brain cholinesterase, serum alkaline phosphatase, and the histopathology of the brain, liver, and kidneys were all investigated but no effects were found (Canton et al., 1975).

When guppies *(Poecilia reticulata)* aged 3-4 weeks were exposed to 0, 200, 800, or 2000 µg alpha-HCH (> 95%) per litre in a 50-day study, the EC_{50}, based on mortality and immobilization, was 800 (600-1200) µg/litre (Canton et al., 1975).

In a study by Janssen et al. (1987), fertilized eggs of *Oryzia latipes* were exposed for 35 days (up to 28 days after hatching) to alpha-HCH. No influence on growth, mortality or behaviour was seen at 800 µg/litre.

9.5 Terrestrial organisms

No data on terrestrial organisms are available.

Table 5. Acute toxicity (48 h) of alpha-hexachlorocyclohexane for fish (growth inhibition/mortality or immobilization)

Species	Age	Temperature (°C)	Parameter	Concentration (mg/litre)	References
Freshwater					
Poecilia reticulata	3-4 weeks	24	EC_{50}^a	0.8 (0.6-1.2)	Canton et al. (1975)
Salmo gairdneri	4 weeks	12	EC_{50}^a	1.05 (0.9-1.2)	Canton et al. (1975)
Saltwater[a]					
Poecilia reticulata	3 weeks	24	EC_{50}^b	1.38 (1.35-1.42)	Canton et al. (1978)
Poecilia reticulata			LC_{50}	3.5	Boulekbache (1980)

[a] closed system
[b] water renewal system

PART B

ENVIRONMENTAL HEALTH CRITERIA

FOR

BETA-HEXACHLOROCYCLOHEXANE

CONTENTS

ENVIRONMENTAL HEALTH CRITERIA FOR
BETA-HEXACHLOROCYCLOHEXANE

1. SUMMARY AND EVALUATION   71

   1.1 General properties   71
   1.2 Environmental transport, distribution, and
        transformation   71
   1.3 Environmental levels and human exposure   71
   1.4 Kinetics and metabolism   73
   1.5 Effects on organisms in the environment   74
   1.6 Effects on experimental animals and
        in vitro test systems   74
   1.7 Effects on humans   75

2. IDENTITY, PHYSICAL AND CHEMICAL
   PROPERTIES, ANALYTICAL METHODS   76

   2.1 Identity of primary constituent   76
   2.2 Physical and chemical properties   76
   2.3 Analytical methods   77

3. SOURCES OF HUMAN AND ENVIRONMENTAL
   EXPOSURE   78

4. ENVIRONMENTAL TRANSPORT, DISTRIBUTION,
   AND TRANSFORMATION   79

   4.1 Transport and distribution between media   79
   4.2 Biotransformation and bioaccumulation   80
        4.2.1 Biodegradation   80
        4.2.2 Abiotic degradation   81
        4.2.3 Bioaccumulation   81
               4.2.3.1 Aquatic invertebrates   81
               4.2.3.2 Fish   82
               4.2.3.3 Birds   82
               4.2.3.4 Bioaccumulation in humans   83
   4.3 Isomerization   83

5. ENVIRONMENTAL LEVELS AND HUMAN EXPOSURE   84

    5.1   Environmental levels   84
           5.1.1   Air   84
           5.1.2   Water   84
                 5.1.2.1   Fresh water   84
                 5.1.2.2   Sea water   85
           5.1.3   Soil/sediment   85
                 5.1.3.1   Dumping grounds   85
           5.1.4   Food and feed   86
           5.1.5   Terrestrial and aquatic organisms   88
                 5.1.5.1   Aquatic organism   88
                 5.1.5.2   Birds   88
                 5.1.5.3   Mammals   89
    5.2   General population exposure   89
           5.2.1   Total-diet studies   90
           5.2.2   Concentrations in human samples   91
                 5.2.2.1   Blood   91
                 5.2.2.2   Adipose tissue   92
                 5.2.2.3   Breast milk   94

6. KINETICS AND METABOLISM   97

    6.1   Absorption and elimination   97
    6.2   Distribution   97
    6.3   Transplacental transfer and transfer via lactation   98
    6.4   Metabolic transformation   99
           6.4.1   Rat   99
           6.4.2   Mouse   99
           6.4.3   Human   100

7. EFFECTS ON LABORATORY MAMMALS AND
IN VITRO TEST SYSTEMS   101

    7.1   Acute toxicity data   101
           7.1.1   Oral   101
           7.1.2   Intraperitoneal   101
    7.2   Short-term exposure   101
           7.2.1   Mouse oral studies   101
           7.2.2.   Rat oral studies   102
    7.3   Skin and eye irritation; sensitization   103

7.4	Long-term exposure		104
	7.4.1	Rat oral studies	104
7.5	Reproduction, embryotoxicity, and teratogenicity		104
	7.5.1	Reproduction	104
	7.5.2	Teratogenicity	105
7.6	Mutagenicity and related end-points		105
7.7	Carcinogenicity		106
	7.7.1	Mouse	106
	7.7.2	Rat	107
	7.7.3	Initiation-promotion	107
	7.7.4	Mode of action	108
7.8	Special studies		109
	7.8.1	Effects on endocrine organs	109
	7.8.2	Neurotoxicity	109
	7.8.3	Effect on liver enzymes	110
	7.8.4	Immunosuppression	111

8. **EFFECTS ON HUMANS** — 112

8.1	Acute toxicity - poisoning incidents	112
8.2	General population	112
8.3	Occupational exposure	112

9. **EFFECTS ON OTHER ORGANISMS IN THE LABORATORY AND FIELD** — 115

9.1	Algae		115
9.2	Protozoa		115
9.3	Invertebrates		115
9.4	Fish		116
	9.4.1	Acute toxicity	116
	9.4.2	Longer-term toxicity	116
9.5	Terrestrial organisms		117
	9.5.1	Birds	117
9.6	Model ecosystem studies		117

1. SUMMARY AND EVALUATION

1.1 General properties

Beta-hexachlorocyclohexane (beta-HCH) is a by-product (7-10%) in the manufacture of lindane (> 99% gamma-HCH). Its solubility in water is low, but it is very soluble in organic solvents such as acetone, cyclohexane, and xylene. It is a solid with a low vapour pressure. The n-octanol/water partition coefficient (log P_{ow}) is 3.80. It is an environmental pollutant.

Beta-HCH can be determined separately from the other isomers by gas chromatography with electron capture detection and other methods after extraction by liquid/liquid partition and purification by column chromatography.

1.2 Environmental transport, distribution, and transformation

Biodegradation and abiotic degradation (dechlorination) by ultraviolet irradiation occur in the environment and produce pentachlorocyclohexane, but at a much slower rate than in the case of lindane (gamma-HCH).

Beta-HCH is the most persistent HCH isomer. Its persistence in soil is determined by environmental factors such as the action of microorganisms, content of organic matter and water, and co-distillation and evaporation from soil.

Owing to the persistence of beta-HCH, rapid bioconcentration takes place in invertebrates (the bioconcentration factor is approximately 125 within 3 days), fish (250-1500 on a dry weight basis or approximately 500 000 times on a lipid basis within 3-10 days), birds and man (approximately 525). The bioconcentration is higher and the elimination is slower for beta-HCH than for the other HCH isomers.

1.3 Environmental levels and human exposure

Beta-HCH is found in air over the oceans at a concentration of 0.004-0.13 ng/m^3.

Summary and Evaluation

Until 1974, the River Rhine and its tributaries contained beta-HCH levels of 0.14-0.22 µg/litre, but thereafter the levels were consistently below 0.1 µg per litre. Samples from the River Meuse also contained < 0.1 µg/litre. In the River Elbe, levels decreased from an average of 0.009 to 0.004 µg/litre between 1981 and 1988.

Beta-HCH has been measured in birds such as sparrowhawks, kestrels, owls, herons, and grebe over a number of years and the concentrations ranged from 0.1 to 0.3 mg/kg. Up to 0.87 mg/kg (on a fat basis) has been found in the liver and adipose tissue of the polar bear.

Important food items have been analysed in a few countries for the presence of beta-HCH. The mean concentrations, mainly in fat-containing food products, ranged up to 0.03 mg/kg (on a fat basis), but in milk products levels up to 4 mg/kg (on a fat basis) were found. In non-fatty food items, the levels were < 0.005 mg/kg product. In general, levels are slowly decreasing.

Food is the main source for general population exposure to beta-HCH. In total-diet studies in the United Kingdom, 0.003, 0.0005, and < 0.0005 mg/kg were found for the years 1966-1967, 1975-1977, and 1981, respectively. In the USA, the average daily intake of beta-HCH in 1982-1984 ranged from < 0.1-0.4 ng/kg body weight for various age groups.

In a number of countries, the concentration of beta-HCH has been determined in the blood, serum, or plasma of the general population. The concentrations varied between the different countries and ranged up to 25 µg/litre.

Many studies have been carried out to determine the presence of beta-HCH in human adipose tissues. The concentrations found in Canada, Germany, Kenya, the Netherlands, and the United Kingdom ranged up to 4.4 mg/kg (on a fat basis). A gradual increase with age was found up to approximately 50 years; thereafter levels decreased. Beta-HCH concentrations in adipose tissues are higher than those of the other HCH isomers, a phenomenon that reflects the accumulative properties of beta-HCH. There is, in general, no clear trend for a decrease in beta-HCH concentrations over the period that studies have been made.

There is a relationship between the concentrations in adipose tissue and breast milk and the consumption of meat products, animal fat, and fatty fish.

In a few countries (Canada, Germany, the Netherlands, and the United Kingdom), breast milk has been analysed and beta-HCH levels of between 0.1 and 0.69 mg/kg (on a fat basis) have been found. The levels in the milk of women living in rural areas appears to be higher than in urban areas.

The high beta-HCH levels that have been found in breast milk exceed permissible concentrations temporarily and locally. The beta-HCH concentrations in the blood of babies lie within the same range as those in the mothers.

Beta-HCH appears to be a universal environmental contaminant. Concentrations are only decreasing very slowly in spite of measures taken to prevent its spread into the environment.

1.4 Kinetics and metabolism

Up to 95% of beta-HCH in the mouse gastrointestinal tract is absorbed, most of it being subsequently accumulated in adipose tissue. The elimination follows a 2-stage mechanism, the half-life for the first stage being 2.5 days and for the second stage 18 days.

After absorption, beta-HCH is rapidly distributed to the liver, brain, kidneys, and adipose tissues. The maximum concentration in the liver is reached in rats after 4 days. At an average blood concentration of 92 μg/litre (but also with concentrations of 540 and 2100 μg per litre), the brain to blood and adipose tissue to blood ratios were 2:1 and 170:1, respectively. After lethal acute human poisoning with HCH isomers, the beta-HCH concentration, relative to that of blood, was 363 in fat, 3 in the brain, and 15 in the liver. Beta-HCH passes the blood-brain barrier much less readily than the other HCH isomers.

Transplacental transfer from pregnant mice to their fetuses was about 2% of the dose, but in rats a transfer of 40% was found. Lactational transfer in rats from dams to sucklings via milk was about 60% of the dose.

In rats 70% of beta-HCH is eliminated during 28 days, one third of this being excreted in the urine. No unchanged beta-HCH is present in the urine. The major metabolite resulting from cis-dehydrochlorination is 2,4,6-trichlorophenol in a conjugated form.

Pretreatment with beta-HCH alters the metabolism of lindane in rats. From intraperitoneal studies with mice, it seems that beta-HCH is metabolized more slowly than lindane.

1.5 Effects on organisms in the environment

Beta-HCH generally has moderate toxicity for algae, invertebrates, and fish. The acute LD_{50} values for these organisms are of the order of 1 mg/litre, but the EC_{50} values are lower (0.05-0.5 mg/litre). The no-observed-effect level for *Oryzia latipes* and *Poecilia reticulata*, two freshwater fish exposed for 1 or 3 months, was 0.03 mg/litre.

No data are available on effects on populations and ecosystems.

1.6 Effects on experimental animals and *in vitro* test systems

The acute oral LD_{50} values for mice and rats were reported in 1968 to lie between 1500 and 2000 mg/kg body weight. However, more recent studies yielded values of 16 g/kg body weight for mice and 8 g/kg body weight for rats. Signs of intoxication were mainly of neurological origin.

Two short-term mouse studies, with dose levels of up to 600 mg/kg diet for 26-32 weeks, showed increased liver weight and nodular hyperplasia and atypical proliferations in the liver. In a third study, dose levels of up to 500 mg/kg diet for 24 weeks did not result in liver tumours or nodular hyperplasia.

A 90-day study with rats fed 50 or 250 mg/kg diet revealed liver changes, i.e. hypertrophy and proliferation of smooth endoplasmic reticulum and increased activity of microsomal enzymes. Changes in the gonads occurred at the highest dose levels but these were associated with severe effects on body weight. Hormonal changes associated with the gonadal atrophy showed no consistent endocrine effect. There were no adverse effects at a dose level of 2 mg/kg diet (equivalent to 0.1 mg/kg body weight).

In a long-term rat study (reported in 1950), doses of 10 mg/kg diet (equivalent to 0.5 mg/kg body weight) or more led to liver enlargement and histological changes.

In a two-generation reproduction study on rats, the same effects were found as in the 90-day study. There were no effects at 2 mg/kg diet (equivalent to 0.1 mg/kg body weight), but a dose level of 10 mg/kg diet resulted in increased mortality and infertility. No compound-related teratogenic effects were found in an extension to this study.

A weak "estrogenic" effect has been described. The uterus was the target organ for this effect; there were no clear effects on endocrine control systems. The mechanism and significance of this effect are uncertain.

The mutagenicity studies reported did not show any increase in mutation frequency in *Salmonella typhimurium* strains. An *in vivo* bone marrow metaphase analysis in rats yielded positive results.

Two studies have been carried out on mice to determine carcinogenic potential. In one study, 200 mg/kg diet was given for 110 weeks, and liver enlargement, hyperplastic changes, and an increase in benign and malignant tumours were reported. In the other study, where 500 mg/kg diet was administered for 24 weeks, no tumours were observed.

Studies in which rats were fed combinations of beta-HCH with polychlorinated biphenyls suggested a promoting effect of beta-HCH.

At 300 mg/kg diet, beta-HCH caused significant changes in several immune functions in mice within one month.

1.7 Effects on humans

When workers at a lindane-producing factory, with a geometric mean exposure of 7.2 years (1-30), were investigated, it was concluded that occupational HCH exposure did not induce signs of neurological impairment or perturbation of "neuromuscular function".

2. IDENTITY, PHYSICAL AND CHEMICAL PROPERTIES, ANALYTICAL METHODS

2.1 Identity of primary constituent

Common name   Beta-hexachlorocyclohexane (beta-HCH)

Chemical formula $C_6H_6Cl_6$

Chemical structure (see Annex I)   Beta-HCH is a stereoisomer of gamma-HCH, the active ingredient of lindane (> 99% gamma-HCH). It differs in the spatial orientation of the hydrogen and chlorine atoms on the carbon atoms:

Relative molecular mass   290.9

CAS chemical name $1\alpha,2\beta,3\alpha,4\beta,5\alpha,6\beta$-hexachlorocyclohexane

Common synonym   Beta-benzenehexachloride (beta-BHC)

CAS registry number   319-85-7

RTECS registry number   GV4375000

2.2 Physical and chemical properties

Some physical and chemical properties are summarized in Table 6.

Table 6. Some physical and chemical properties of beta-hexachlorocyclohexane

Melting point	309 °C
Vapour pressure (20 °C)	0.67 Pa (0.005 mmHg)
Relative density (20 °C)	1.89 g/cm^3
Solubility	
water (20 °C)	1.5 mg/litre
water (28 °C)	0.2 mg/litre
organic solvents (20 °C)	
acetone	103.9 g/litre
chloroform	3 g/litre
ethanol	11 g/litre
petroleum ether	1-2 g/litre
xylene	33 g/litre
cyclohexane	121 g/litre
Stability	considerable stability in acids, unstable in alkaline conditions
n-Octanol/water partition coefficient (log P_{ow})	3.80

2.3 Analytical methods

The same methods can be used as for alpha-HCH (see section 2.3 alpha-HCH).

3. SOURCES OF HUMAN AND ENVIRONMENTAL EXPOSURE

Beta-HCH does not occur naturally. It is released to the environment as a result of the use of technical-grade HCH and the inappropriate disposal of the residue resulting from the purification of lindane.

Beta-HCH is basically a by-product (and impurity) in the manufacturing of lindane (> 99% gamma-HCH) (van Velsen, 1986). Technical-grade HCH, which is synthesized from benzene and chlorine in the presence of ultraviolet light, consists of:

65-70%	alpha-HCH
7-10%	beta-HCH
14-15%	gamma-HCH (lindane)
≈ 7%	delta-HCH
≈ 1-2%	epsilon-HCH
≈ 1-2%	other components

Purification of lindane produces a residue, consisting almost entirely of non-insecticidal HCH isomers (mainly alpha- and beta-), which can be used as an intermediate for the production of trichlorobenzene and other chemicals.

Alpha- and beta-HCH have been used in mixtures with gamma-HCH (as "HCH" or "fortified HCH") in agriculture and in wood protection.

4. ENVIRONMENTAL TRANSPORT, DISTRIBUTION, AND TRANSFORMATION

4.1 Transport and distribution between media

Tsukano (1973) studied the factors affecting the disappearance of beta-HCH from rice field soil. After granular application of technical-grade HCH (0.05 mg/litre) into surface water, beta-HCH disappeared very slowly (half-life > 28 days). After the translocation of beta-HCH (1 mg/litre) onto flooded levelled soil, the surface water and soil was analysed at intervals. A decrease in the beta-HCH concentration in water and a steady increase in soil was found. After 7 days a maximum concentration in soil was reached. From a soil column study it was found that beta-HCH did not move through the soil.

Suzuki et al. (1975) studied the persistence of beta-HCH in three different types of soils. Beta-HCH is the most persistent isomer of HCH, the persistence being dependent on environmental factors such as the action of soil microorganisms, co-distillation, and evaporation from soil. Furthermore, the water content and the content of organic matter in the soil are of importance.

Siddaramappa & Sethunathan (1975) studied the persistence of ^{14}C-labelled beta-HCH in five Indian rice soils under flooded conditions, using incubation times of 0, 20, and 41 days. The degradation of beta-HCH was much slower than that of lindane. However, there was a great difference in the degradation rates between the soils. In two types of soils (sandy and kari soils) both isomers persisted even after 41 days of flooding.

Sorption and desorption of beta-HCH by 12 soils from rice-growing areas in India were studied using a ^{14}C-label. The soils showed striking differences in their ability to adsorb beta-HCH, the sorption values ranging from 46 to 96% of total added beta-HCH. After oxidation of the soil with hydrogen peroxide, the sorption was lower (14-58%). Organic matter was the most important factor governing the sorption and desorption, but pH, exchange acidity, exchangeable sodium and magnesium, and electrical conductivity also affected the results (Wahid & Sethunathan, 1979).

Kampe (1980) concluded from experimental data that the transport of beta-HCH to ground water is unlikely, owing to low water solubility and anaerobic degradation.

Korte (1980) summarized the behaviour of beta-HCH in the environment, especially in soil and plants.

4.2 Biotransformation and bioaccumulation

4.2.1 Biodegradation

MacRae et al. (1967) studied the persistence and biodegradability of beta-HCH in two clay soils. Beta-HCH was applied at a level of 15 mg/kg soil and the incubation periods were 0, 15, 30, 50, 70, and 90 days. In non-sterilized soils only very small amounts could be detected after 70 days, indicating biodegradation, whereas in sterilized soils the losses were much slower and probably due to volatilization.

In studies using either mixed or pure bacterial cultures under anaerobic or aerobic conditions, the dechlorination of ^{36}Cl-labelled beta-HCH by mixed soil flora and by pure cultures of *Citrobacter freundii, C. butyricum,* and *C. pasteurianum* was 7.4, 15.3, 23.8, and 10.1%, respectively, within 6 days of incubation. Aerobically grown facultative anaerobes dechlorinated actively. Beta-HCH degraded more slowly than lindane (Jagnow et al., 1977; Haider, 1979).

Cell suspensions of *Clostridium sphenoides* cultured under anaerobic conditions did not degrade beta-HCH (10 mg/litre) within 24 h. Even with more concentrated cell suspensions of the organism and conditions most conducive to lindane degradation (pH 8.0, 40 °C), there was no indication of any degradation (Heritage & MacRae, 1979).

MacRae et al. (1984) carried out laboratory studies on the transformation of beta-HCH (dosage: 20 mg beta-HCH/g of soil) in a Japanese soil containing 4% organic carbon under both aerobic and anaerobic conditions. From the transformation rates, half-life values of 91 and 122 days, respectively, were calculated.

In a study by Doelman et al. (1988a), microbial soil sanitation was applied to calcareous alkaline sandy loam soil that was polluted with a mixture of HCH isomers. Under anaerobic conditions, microbial degradation in the Dutch climate (soil temperature of 5-17 °C) did not occur, and even the low concentration of the easily degradable gamma-HCH did not decrease. Microbial soil sanitation of beta-HCH-polluted sandy loam soil systems have been investigated. The soil systems involved were aerated moist soil and continuously aerated and intermittently aerated thick soil slurry. Degradation of beta-HCH did not take place during a 40-week incubation period (Doelman et al., 1988b).

A field investigation into the distribution of HCHs was carried out by Chessells et al. (1988) using soil from an agricultural area treated with BHC-20 (HCH composition: 70% alpha-HCH, 6.5% beta-HCH, 13.5% gamma-HCH, and 5% delta-HCH. The beta-HCH concentration decreased only very slowly, probably owing to its comparatively high stability and low water solubility. Furthermore, soil organic carbon content was found to be of primary importance. A significant decrease in isomer concentration was observed when soil moisture content was high and was attributed to microbial degradation favoured by these conditions.

4.2.2 Abiotic degradation

Ultraviolet irradiation, using a 15-watt low pressure mercury lamp, of beta-HCH in 2-propanol solution for 16 h resulted in the production of an isomer of pentachlorocyclohexene. This substance seems to be formed by the migration of an equatorial chlorine atom to the vicinal axial position at the intermediate pentachlorocyclohexyl radical (Hamada et al., 1982).

4.2.3 Bioaccumulation

4.2.3.1 Aquatic invertebrates

In a study by Yamato et al. (1983), short-necked clam *(Venerupis japonica)* rapidly absorbed beta-HCH and the concentration reached a plateau on the third day. The bioconcentration factor was 127 at a beta-HCH concentration in water of 2 µg/litre. The beta-HCH concentrations on day 6 in internal organs and tissues were 0.194 and 0.076 mg/kg, respectively. After a 3-day elimination period, the levels were 0.115 and 0.075 mg/kg, respectively.

4.2.3.2 Fish

Sugiura et al. (1979) studied bioaccumulation in the carp *(Cyprinus carpio)*, brown trout *(Salmo trutta fario)*, golden orfe *(Leuciscus idus melanotus)*, and guppy *(Poecilia reticulata)*. Beta-HCH was dissolved in water to a concentration of 1 mg/litre under steady-state conditions (time period not specified), and the equilibrium bioconcentration factors for the four types of fish were 273, 658, 973, and 1485, respectively.

In a study by Yamato et al. (1983), guppies *(Poecilia reticulata)* rapidly bioaccumulated beta-HCH and the tissue concentration reached a plateau on the fourth day. The beta-HCH concentration in the water was 2 µg/litre and the bioconcentration factor 1043. The concentration in the guppy slowly decreased on the first day after the fish were transferred to HCH-free water.

In general, the equilibrium levels were reached within 3-10 days. A bioconcentration factor of 100 000 to 500 000 has been calculated using data on the concentration of beta-HCH in the muscle and fat of bream collected in the River Elbe (Arbeitsgemeinschaft für die Reinhaltung der Elbe, 1982).

4.2.3.3 Birds

When low levels of HCH were administered together with other organochloropesticides in the feed to broilers for 6-16 weeks, of the three HCH isomers tested (alpha, beta, and gamma), beta-HCH showed the greatest bioaccumulation (the mean bioconcentration factors for eggs and fat were 13 and 15, respectively). The half-life (after administration of uncontaminated food for 12 weeks) was about 6-8 weeks (Kan & Jonker-den Rooyen, 1978a,b; Kan et al., 1978).

This relatively higher accumulation of beta-HCH was also observed in chickens after feeding diets fortified with 1 mg beta-HCH/kg for 4 weeks. The order of the degradation rate for the four HCH isomers was delta > gamma >

alpha > beta. Biotransformation to one or more of the other HCH isomers did not occur (Szokolay et al., 1977a).

4.2.3.4 Bioaccumulation in humans

Geyer et al. (1986) found that in industrialized countries more than 90% of the non-occupation exposure to HCHs derives from food. The mean concentration (on a fat basis) of beta-HCH in human adipose tissue was found to be 0.33-0.38, 0.40, 0.31, 0.90, 0.27, and 0.31 mg/kg in the Federal Republic of Germany, the Netherlands, USSR, Switzerland, USA, and United Kingdom, respectively. The mean bioconcentration factor (on a lipid basis), calculated on the basis of the concentration in the diet (0.68, 0.62, 1.0, 1.21, 0.56, and 0.67 µg/kg, respectively) and the levels in adipose tissue, was 527.0 ± 140 (range 310-744).

4.3 Isomerization

Deo et al. (1980, 1981) studied the isomerization of beta-HCH by shaking it with distilled water at 25 °C for various time intervals (5 min to 4 days). The results of GLC analysis of the extracts indicated that a small portion of the beta-HCH isomerized into alpha-, gamma-, and delta-HCH. There were indications that other compounds were also formed by reactions such as dehydrochlorination. Toxicity studies with mosquito larvae, flour beetle larvae, and houseflies exposed to the extracts demonstrated that the resulting aqueous solution contained substances that were more toxic than beta-HCH.

5. ENVIRONMENTAL LEVELS AND HUMAN EXPOSURE

5.1 Environmental levels

5.1.1 Air

Tanabe et al. (1982) found an average of 0.03 ng beta-HCH/m^3 (0.004-0.13 ng/m^3) in 24 samples of air over the Western Pacific, Eastern Indian, and Antarctic Oceans.

The concentrations of beta-HCH measured in the air of Delft, the Netherlands, in 1979-1980 were below the limit of detection (2-3 pg/m^3) (Slooff & Matthijsen, 1988).

5.1.2 Water

5.1.2.1 Fresh water

During the period 1969-1977, 1826 water samples were taken at 99 sampling sites in the Netherlands. The highest concentrations of beta-HCH were found in the River Rhine and its tributaries. The concentrations during the period 1969-1974 were 0.14-0.22 µg/litre, but from 1974 on, the concentrations were all below 0.1 µg/litre. A sampling trip by boat made along the River Rhine from Rheinfelden in Switzerland to Rotterdam in the Netherlands proved that the source of alpha-, beta-, and gamma-HCH was located in the upper Rhine. In the River Meuse, the levels were all below 0.1 µg/litre during the period 1969-1977 (Wegman & Greve, 1980). Since 1983 the contents of beta-HCH in the Rivers Rhine, Meuse, and West-Scheldt and in other surface waters in the Netherlands have generally been below 0.001 µg/litre (Slooff & Matthijsen, 1988). The average concentration of dissolved beta-HCH in the Meuse-Rhine estuary in 1974 was 6 ng/litre whereas that of suspended beta-HCH was < 1 to 3 ng/litre (Slooff & Matthijsen, 1988).

The Arbeitsgemeinschaft der Elbe (the Elbe Study Group) investigated the presence of beta-HCH in the River Elbe from Schnackenburg to the North Sea in 1981-1982 and found a mean concentration of 0.009 (< 0.001-0.072) µg per litre. During the period February to November 1988 the concentrations varied from 0.001 to 0.009 µg per litre (Arbeitsgemeinschaft der Elbe, 1988).

In the surface water of the Upper Rhine, the beta-HCH concentration was 200 ng/litre in 1974 but decreased in 1976-1977 to 2-25 ng/litre (Hildebrandt et al., 1986). LWA (1987) failed to detect beta-HCH in the River Rhine (three locations) and in six tributaries.

5.1.2.2 *Sea water*

Beta-HCH was detected in the North Sea at a level of 1.4 µg/litre in 1972 (Mestres, 1974), but in June-July 1986 the levels in surface water (5 m) were < 0.03-0.2 ng/litre (Umweltbundesamt, 1989).

The concentration of beta-HCH in the Japan Sea and the Pacific Ocean around Japan was below the detection limit of 0.1 µg/litre in 1974 (personal communications by A. Hamada and by T. Onishi to the IPCS, July 1989).

5.1.3 *Soil/sediment*

In 1974 beta-HCH was found in 9 out of 60 sediment samples collected in Japan, the range of concentration being 30-50 µg/kg (personal communications by A. Hamada and by T. Onishi to the IPCS, July 1989).

Slooff & Matthijsen (1988) analysed sediments from eight different locations close to dumping places in the Netherlands for the presence of alpha-, beta-, and gamma-HCH and obtained median values for beta-HCH of 9-214 µg per kg dry matter.

5.1.3.1 *Dumping grounds*

In the Netherlands soil has been polluted with HCHs at various location as the result of their manufacture in the 1950s (spillage during production, storage, and handling), and concentrations up to a few grams of HCHs/kg dry soil have been found. Further pollution has been caused by both the dumping of chemical waste and its use in the levelling of certain areas. From these dumping areas dispersal of the chemical waste can occur by leaching or wind erosion from open storage depots. In certain polluted areas, high concentrations of HCHs, mainly the alpha and beta-isomers, have been found more than 2 m below ground level. In 18 locations in the Netherlands, the average concentrations of beta-HCH in sewage sludge in 1981 were between 30 and 150 µg/kg dry matter. Pollution of ground water also occurred, but this was restricted to the vicinity of the production areas. Horizontal transportation of HCHs in ground water appeared to be limited (Slooff & Matthijsen, 1988).

5.1.4 Food and feed

The concentration of beta-HCH has been determined in a number of important food items in France. The mean concentration was 0.03 (nd-0.25) mg/kg in milk and milk products (2688 samples), 0.02 (nd-0.04) mg/kg in meat (27 samples), 0.01 (nd-0.03) mg/kg in meat products (34 samples), and 0.01 (nd-0.1) mg/kg in animal fat (67 samples). In other food items, beta-HCH was not detected (< 0.005 mg/kg) (Laugel, 1981).

In a survey of milk contamination carried out in various areas of Japan in 1970, the average beta-HCH content in cow's milk ranged from 0.009 mg/litre in the Hokkaido area to 1.288 mg/litre in the Nagasaki area (Matsushima, 1972).

Table 7 gives the mean beta-HCH levels in a large number of samples of various food items from the Federal Republic of Germany reported by Hildebrandt et al. (1986).

Skaftason & Johannesson (1979) analysed a total of 32 samples of butter from Iceland between 1974 and 1978 and found beta-HCH, at a mean concentration of 23 ± 16 µg per kg, in 31 out of 32 samples.

In six samples of cow's milk collected from six locations in Switzerland, the levels of beta-HCH were 1.0-4.0 mg/kg on a fat basis (Rappe et al., 1987).

In a study carried out in the United Kingdom, 24 samples of each food group were analysed. Bread, other cereal products, meat products, fish, oils and fats, eggs, green vegetables, potatoes, other vegetables, and fresh fruit contained no detectable amounts of beta-HCH. Carcass meat contained < 0.0005 (nd-0.003) mg/kg, offals < 0.0005 (nd-0.003) mg/kg, poultry 0.008 (nd-0.08) mg/kg, milk < 0.0005 (nd-0.001) mg/kg, and dairy products 0.001

Table 7. Beta-hexachlorocyclohexane concentrations (mg/kg) in various food items[a]

Food items	1973-78	1979-83	1973-83
Meat[b]		0.01-0.083 (0.26)[d]	
Meat products[b]		0.003-0.055 (0.15)[d]	
Animal fat[b]			0.003-0.024 (0.075)[d]
Game[b]			0.025-0.285
Poultry[b]		0.001-0.016 (0.42)[d]	
Chicken eggs			0.001
Fish		0.001-0.007	
Milk and milk products[b]	0.05	< 0.01	
Butter[b,c]		< 0.01-0.02	
Cereals			up to 0.001
Cereal products			up to 0.01

[a] From: Hildebrandt et al. (1986).
[b] Determinations made on a fat basis
[c] Anon (1984)
[d] maximum value

(nd-0.008) mg/kg. Imported meat products collected in 1981-1983 contained up to 1.4 mg/kg product, imported retail cereal products collected in 1982 contained up to 0.03 mg/kg and animal feed collected in 1984 contained up to 0.08 mg/kg (HMSO, 1986).

No beta-HCH was found in meat and poultry products including eggs (976 samples) collected during 1984-1986. Peanut butter and vegetable oils (in total 95 samples) showed mean beta-HCH levels of 0.01-0.02 mg/kg product, whereas processed pork and poultry products collected in 1985-1987 contained mean levels of 0.2 and 1.9 mg/kg, respectively. Twenty-six out of 86 samples were positive and the highest level that was found was 6.3 mg/kg. Other processed meat products (631 samples) contained up to 0.01 mg/kg product. In 1984-1987, retail milk and dairy products were analysed, and 499 out of 849 samples contained beta-HCH at a mean concentration of 0.01-0.03 mg/kg product (the highest level was 0.08 mg/kg). Samples of eel muscle (1124 eels from 62 sites) collected during 1986-1987 showed mean beta-HCH concentration of up to 0.02 mg/kg. The highest level found was 0.05 mg/kg (HMSO, 1989).

5.1.5 Terrestrial and aquatic organisms

5.1.5.1 Aquatic organism

Mouvet et al. (1985) measured the presence of beta-HCH in the aquatic moss *Cinclidotus danubicus* in order to examine its potential use as an indicator of chlorinated pollutants in fresh water. The level in water 4 km downstream of an industrial discharge was 0.5-2.6 µg per litre, while the levels in moss 0, 13, 24, and 51 days after transplant to the polluted river were < 0.025, 0.025-0.33, 0.025-1.29, and 0.4 mg/kg dry weight, respectively.

Bream collected from various locations in the River Elbe (between Schnackenburg and the North Sea) contained beta-HCH levels of 0.008-0.063 mg/kg in muscle tissue and 0.7-2.8 mg/kg in adipose tissue (Arbeitsgemeinschaft für die Reinhaltung der Elbe, 1982).

Freshwater fish from different rivers in the Federal Republic of Germany were analysed during the period 1973-1981. In the first 3-4 years the beta-HCH levels were mainly between 0.01-0.02 mg/kg fresh weight. However, a decrease then took place and most of the samples were below 0.01 mg/kg fresh weight, with the exception of certain types of fish such as the eel and fish from industrially contaminated areas. In 1981-1983, shell-fish and molluscs were analysed in the Federal Republic of Germany, and the beta-HCH concentration ranged from < 0.001 to 0.011 mg/kg fresh weight (Hildebrandt et al., 1986).

5.1.5.2 Birds

Organochlorine pesticides were determined in the livers of predatory birds in the United Kingdom during

1963-1966. The average residues (arithmetic means) of beta-HCH found are given in Table 8.

Table 8. Residues of beta-hexachlorocyclohexane in the livers of predatory birds[a]

Species	Year	Number of samples	Concentration (mg/kg)
Sparrowhawk	1963	11	0.3
	1964	8	0.23
	1965	9	0.25
Kestrel	1964	28	0.1
	1965	60	0.01
Tawny owl	1963	12	0.02
	1965	29	0.01
Barn owl	1964	23	0.07
Heron (adults)	1964	17	0.1
Heron (nestlings)	1965	20	0.005
Great crested grebe	1963/1966	15	0.1

[a] From: HMSO (1969)

5.1.5.3 Mammals

Skaftason & Johannesson (1979) analysed samples of body fat from 10-year-old sheep, collected in 1974 in Iceland, and found an average of 79 ± 48 µg beta-HCH/kg.

Norström et al. (1988) determined the contamination of Canadian arctic and subarctic marine ecosystems by analysing the adipose tissue and liver of polar bears *(Ursus maritimus;* 6-20 animals per area) collected from 12 areas between 1982-1984. Of the total HCH in adipose tissue, 29% was beta-HCH (0.3-0.87 mg/kg on a fat basis).

5.2 General population exposure

From the data presented in section 5.1 it is evident that food is the main source of exposure of the general population to beta-HCH.

5.2.1 Total-diet studies

In a total-diet study carried out in the United Kingdom during 1966-1985, food purchased in 21 towns throughout the country was prepared by cooking. The study covered 20 to 24 food groups, and the number of total-diet samples examined varied from 22 to 25 samples. The calculated mean beta-HCH residue levels in the total diet for the periods 1966-1967, 1970-1971, 1974-1975, 1975-1977, 1979-1980, 1981, and 1984-1985 were 0.003, 0.001, 0.0005, 0.005, 0.001, < 0.0005, and < 0.0006 mg/kg, respectively (Egan & Hubbard, 1975; HMSO, 1982, 1986, 1989).

Samples consisting of 50 items of infant food and 110 items of toddler food were collected in 1978-1979 in 10 USA cities. The daily intake of beta-HCH in 1977, 1978, and 1979 in infant food was below the limit of detection. In toddler food beta-HCH was only detectable in 1977, the daily intake being 0.002 µg/kg body weight per day (Gartrell et al., 1985b).

Total-diet studies conducted by the FDA in the USA before 1982 were based on a "composite sample approach" regardless of the diet involved. Later on they were based on dietary survey information and allowed the "total diet" of the population to be represented by a relatively small number of food items for a greater number of age-sex groups. The daily intakes of beta-HCH during 1982-1984 for the age groups 6-11 months, 2 years, 14-16-year-old females, 14-16-year-old males, 25-30-year-old females, 25-30-year-old males, 60-65-year-old females and 60-65-year-old males were < 0.1, 0.3, 0.2, 0.2, 0.2, 0.4, 0.2, and 0.2 ng/kg body weight, respectively (Gunderson, 1988).

Matsushima (1972) reported that the total diet of an average citizen of Matsuyama City, Japan, contained about 0.177 mg HCH/day, the major portion being the beta isomer. Of the beta-HCH intake 90% was identified as originating from meat and dairy products.

In a total-diet study in the Netherlands in 1977, the average concentration of beta-HCH in 100 samples was < 0.02 mg/kg on a fat basis. The highest level was 0.19 mg/kg (Greve & van Hulst, 1977).

5.2.2 Concentrations in human samples

Beta-HCH concentrations in human samples are a good indication of the total exposure of the general population. Concentrations in human tissues are markedly higher than those of the other HCH isomers, a phenomenon which reflects the cumulative properties of the beta isomer. There has been a trend, but only a very slow one, towards lower values in recent data.

Greve (1985) was unable to detect any correlation between life style, such as type of food, and the beta-HCH concentrations in tissues of Dutch citizens. However, in a Swedish study the levels of beta-HCH (and of other organochlorine contaminants) in breast milk were found to be related to dietary habit. Levels in lacto-vegetarians were lower than those in women eating a mixed diet, and the latter were in turn lower than those in women using a mixed diet that regularly included fatty fish from the Baltic (Noren, 1983).

5.2.2.1 Blood

Eckenhausen et al. (1981) detected beta-HCH at a concentration of < 0.5 to 25 µg/litre in the blood of 19 out of 47 pregnant women in the Netherlands. A concentration range of < 1.0 to 12 µg/litre was found in 30 out of 69 women after they had given birth and beta-HCH was detected in the blood of 17 out of 46 babies (< 1.0 to 6.0 µg/litre).

When Blok et al. (1984) studied the presence of beta-HCH in the blood of 65 healthy Dutch volunteers (34 females and 31 males), beta-HCH was found in approximately half of the volunteers. The median concentration was 0.4 µg/litre (range nd-1.4 µg/litre) in both males and females.

Blood samples of Dutch citizens analysed in 1978, 1980, 1981, and 1982 (70, 48, 127, and 54 samples, respectively), contained 0.3-1.4 µg beta-HCH/litre (Greve & Wegman, 1985).

Polishuk et al. (1970) found beta-HCH in the blood of 24 pregnant women and 23 infants living in Israel. The mean concentrations was 0.5 ± 0.6 µg/litre in the women and 0.3 ± 0.5 µg/litre in the infants.

The average concentrations of beta-HCH in the plasma of five subjects in the USA, who were not occupationally exposed, were 0.83-0.94 µg/litre, and were remarkably consistent throughout the 5 days during which samples were taken (Radomski et al., 1971a).

Starr et al. (1974) analysed the blood of 187 men and 171 women living in Colorado, USA. In men, a mean concentration of 4.9 µg beta-HCH/litre was found in 15 samples, while in women the mean concentration in 7 samples was 10.9 µg/litre (range, 9.0-15.0).

In a 4-year study to assess the exposure of the general population, 6252 blood samples were collected from people (12-74 years of age) living in 64 locations across the USA. Beta-HCH was detected in 13.9% of the samples at a mean level of 1.7 µg/litre (range, 1-28 µg/litre). The percentage of positive samples increased from the youngest to oldest age group (from 3.2 to 26.8%) (Murphy & Harvey, 1985).

Bertram et al. (1980) found a median concentration of 1.32 µg beta-HCH/litre (range, nd-4.81) in whole blood (18 samples) of citizens of the Federal Republic of Germany.

5.2.2.2 *Adipose tissue*

In fifteen samples of adipose tissue from the general population of the Federal Republic of Germany, the median concentration of beta-HCH was 0.33 mg/kg on a fat basis (range, nd-0.66) (Bertram et al., 1980).

Specimens of subcutaneous adipose tissue from 48 children (34 under the age of 1 year, 14 in the second year of life) were analysed during the period 1982-1983 in the Federal Republic of Germany. The average concentration of beta-HCH was 0.15 (range, nd-1.02) mg/kg fat. The average concentration was highest, 0.17 (nd-0.38) mg/kg fat, at the age of 0-6 weeks (Niessen et al., 1984).

Hildebrandt et al. (1986) summarized the results of nine studies carried out in the Federal Republic of Germany in 1969-1983. The mean beta-HCH concentrations

(636 samples) ranged from 0.01 to 1.30 mg/kg on a fat basis.

Mes et al. (1982) analysed 99 samples of adipose tissue from autopsies of accident victims from different areas of Canada. All samples contained beta-HCH, the average concentration of which was 0.151 ± 0.459 (range, 0.016-4.413) mg/kg wet weight. In males (53) the average value was 0.183 ± 0.612 mg/kg, whereas in women (45) it was 0.116 ± 0.166 mg/kg. The influence of age was evident. The average concentration in 33 people aged up to 25 was 0.067 ± 0.051 mg/kg, in 41 people aged 26-50 it was 0.260 ± 0.698 mg/kg, and in 24 people aged 51 or more it was 0.082 ± 0.037 mg/kg.

Human adipose tissue was analysed during the periods 1965-1967, 1969-1971, and 1976-1977 (male and female) in the United Kingdom, the number of samples being 66, 248, 201 (male), and 236 (female), respectively. The arithmetic means of the beta-HCH concentrations were 0.28, 0.27, 0.30 (male), and 0.33 (female) mg/kg, respectively (HMSO, 1982). During 1982-1983, the beta-HCH concentrations were 0.24 (male) and 0.31 (female) with a range of 0.01-0.81 mg/kg (HMSO, 1986).

Kutz et al. (1979) studied the presence of organo-chlorine pesticides in human adipose tissue in 48 states of the USA in 1970-1975. Beta-HCH was widely distributed at low levels (geometric means of between 0.2 and 0.4 mg/kg tissue on a fat basis) during this period, and there was a slow downward trend. Residues of alpha-HCH and gamma-HCH were found at a very low frequency.

In 1980, eight adipose tissue samples were taken as part of the US EPA National Human Monitoring Program in North East Louisiana and in 1984 10 samples were collected. The average beta-HCH concentration (on a lipid basis) was 0.77 mg/kg (nd-2.31) in 1980 and 0.62 mg/kg (0.31-1.03) in 1984 (Holt et al., 1986).

In a study by Szymczynski et al. (1986), 29 samples of adipose tissue were taken at necropsy and 24 at surgery in the Poznan region of Poland and were compared with 100 samples from residents of the Warsaw region. In Poznan, the mean concentration of beta-HCH was 0.211 ± 0.154 mg/kg, while in Warsaw it was 0.184 ± 0.017 mg/kg.

In Kenya, Wassermann et al. (1972) analysed 83 adipose tissue samples collected during autopsy in 1969-1970 from people without occupational exposure to insecticides. The mean concentration of beta-HCH in the age group 5-24 (32 samples) was 0.0686 ± 0.064 mg/kg, in the age group 25-44 (28 samples) it was 0.263 ± 0.266 mg/kg, and in people aged 45 or more (23 samples) it was 0.186 ± 0.228 mg/kg.

In 1974, 360 adipose tissue samples were collected in 8 regions of Japan, and the mean concentration of beta-HCH was 6.55 mg/kg on a fat basis (Takabatake, 1978).

The beta-HCH concentration of 567 samples of adipose tissues of Dutch citizens analysed during 1968-1983 ranged from 0.21 to 0.6 mg/kg (on a fat basis). The highest levels were found in 1968-1976 (Greve & van Harten, 1983; Greve & Wegman, 1985).

5.2.2.3 Breast milk

Breast milk is a major route for the elimination of organochlorine pesticides and PCBs in women. In a study by Cetinkaya et al. (1984), a significant correlation was found between the concentration of beta-HCH in breast milk and the level of consumption of meat products and animal fat. In addition, concentrations of beta-HCH in breast milk in rural areas appeared to be higher than those in urban areas.

The variation during lactation of residue levels in breast milk was investigated in five women aged 23-36 in the Federal Republic of Germany. The beta-HCH concentrations were between 0.04 and 0.20 mg/kg fat, and no significant changes in residue level occurred during the lactation period (Fooken & Butte, 1987).

The residues of beta-HCH in breast milk during the periods 1974-1975 and 1979-1980 in the Federal Republic of Germany were 0.6 and 0.3 mg/kg fat, respectively (Anon., 1984).

More than 7100 samples of breast milk were analysed in the Federal Republic of Germany from 1969 to 1984. These studies were carried out by 20 authors, and the results were summarized by Hildebrandt et al. (1986). The mean concentrations of beta-HCH ranged from 0.02 to 0.56 mg/kg fat. There was no clear decrease in the mean concentrations during the period 1969-1979, but thereafter a slow decrease was observed. A further study carried out in the Federal Republic of Germany (2709 samples in 1979-1981) yielded an average concentration of 0.37 mg/kg fat (Fooken & Butte, 1987). In 1981-1983, 132 samples of breast milk were analysed and the average level was 0.209 mg beta-HCH/kg milk fat (Cetinkaya et al., 1984).

Tuinstra (1971) analysed 42 individual samples of breast milk collected in 1969 from young mothers (18-32 years of age) living in the Netherlands and determined a median beta-HCH concentration of 0.28 mg/kg milk fat (range, 0.1-0.69 mg/kg). When 278 samples of breast milk, collected in 11 maternity centres in the Netherlands, were analysed for the presence of beta-HCH, the median beta-HCH concentration was 0.1 mg/kg (on a fat basis). The maximum value was 0.3 mg/kg (Greve & Wegman, 1985).

Samples of maternal blood, milk, and umbilical cord blood were collected from 43 mothers and their infants during 1981-1982 in Oslo, Norway. The residue levels in maternal and umbilical cord serum were below < 1 µg per kg. In colostrum and milk, concentrations ranging from 0.05 to 0.45 mg/kg fat were found (Skaare et al., 1988).

Vukavic et al. (1986) measured beta-HCH in 59 samples of colostrum collected during autumn 1982 (26 samples) and spring 1983 (33 samples) from healthy nursing mothers on the third day after delivery. The beta-HCH concentrations in the autumn and spring were not significantly different (mean concentrations of 0.95 ± 0.21 and 0.88 ± 0.16 µg/litre whole colostrum, respectively).

Mes et al. (1986) studied 210 breast milk samples from five different regions of Canada and measured a mean beta-HCH concentration of 0.214 mg/kg (on a fat basis). Davies & Mes (1987) studied 18 breast milk samples from Canadian, Indian, and Inuit mothers in Canada, whose fish consumption was comparable to the national consumption. The level of beta-HCH in milk fat of the indigenous population was 0.022 mg/kg, compared with a value of 0.206 mg/kg from a national survey.

In Japan, the average beta-HCH content in breast milk was found to be 0.120 mg/kg (Matsushima, 1972).

In Japan, 378, 328, 87, and 77 samples of breast milk, respectively, were analysed in 1980, 1981, 1982, and 1983. The mean concentrations were 0.031, 0.034, 0.043, and 0.020 mg beta-HCH/kg whole milk, respectively (WHO, 1986).

Breast milk was analysed for the presence of beta-HCH during 1979-1980 and 1983-1984 in the United Kingdom. In these two periods, 30 and 40 samples, respectively, were collected in Scotland. The mean concentrations were 0.008 (< 0.001-0.14) and 0.005 (< 0.001-0.032) mg/kg milk, respectively (HMSO, 1986).

6. KINETICS AND METABOLISM

6.1 Absorption and elimination

Shibata (1978) reported that the absorption of beta-HCH from the gastrointestinal tract in mice was 80-95%, most of this being accumulated in adipose tissue. The elimination followed a 2-stage mechanism, the half-life for the first stage being 2.5 days and that for the second stage being 18 days. The half-life for clearance from blood in rats (sex not specified) was 1 month (Altmann et al., 1980), and the half-life for clearance from fat was 14 days in male rats and 28 days in female rats (Portig, 1983). Vohland & Koransky (1983) reported a half-life for clearance from "internal organs" of 22 days in female rats. A half-life of 20 days for the clearance from the brain of female rats was reported by Portig & Vohland (1983) and Vohland et al. (1981). In cows the half-life for clearance from fat was 4.2-22.0 weeks (Wolf, 1983). The elimination in humans was slow after continuous exposure ceased, the concentration in fatty tissues decreasing only slightly over several years (Vohland & Koransky, 1983).

6.2 Distribution

Oshiba (1972) fed groups of six rats a diet containing 10 mg beta-HCH/kg for up to 56 days. The beta-HCH level in adipose tissue was 60 mg/kg tissue and in the liver was 45 mg/kg tissue after 56 days. The maximum concentration in the liver was reached after 4 weeks. During subsequent starvation, beta-HCH was mobilized from adipose tissue by an enhanced lipid metabolism. Furthermore, there was a tendency for deposition in other organs and tissues.

Vohland et al. (1981) and Portig & Vohland (1983) studied the distribution of beta-HCH in the brain and depot fat of rats. With an average concentration in blood of 92 μg beta-HCH/litre, a brain to blood ratio of 2:1 and depot fat to blood ratio of 170:1 were found, whereas with blood concentrations of 540 μg/litre and 2100 μg per litre the ratios were 2:1 and 177:1 and 2:1 and 168:1, respectively.

After lethal acute intoxication of humans by HCH, the HCH concentration, relative to that in blood, was in the ratio of 363:1 for fat, 3:1 for brain, and 15:1 for liver (Vohland & Koransky, 1983).

When beta-HCH is applied repeatedly to rats, mice, and mini-pigs there is marked storage in fat, especially in females, and the fat levels increase continuously as dosing progresses (Nakajima et al., 1970; Oshiba & Kawakita, 1972; Altmann et al., 1980; van Velsen et al., 1982; Srinivasan & Radhakrishnamurty, 1983). Data on concentrations in organs are contradictory: according to one report the levels in the kidneys, brain, and liver of rats reached a plateau after 4 weeks (Oshiba & Kawakita, 1972), whereas other sources reported steady increases in these organs throughout a 12-week dosing period (van Velsen et al., 1982).

6.3 Transplacental transfer and transfer via lactation

Hori & Kashimoto (1974) found, after oral dosing of pregnant mice, a carry-over from dam to fetus of approximately 2% of the dose. Shibata (1978), however, reported a placental transfer of beta-HCH in rats of approximately 40%.

During lactation the transfer of beta-HCH to milk was 85% from adipose tissue and 64% from administered beta-HCH (Shibata, 1978). Carry-over from dam to suckling via the milk was about 60% of the dose during lactation.

In a study by Hapke & Hollmann (1985), significant carry-over via milk was found after female rats were dosed for a period of 8 weeks that terminated 3 weeks before mating. At both the dose levels tested (i.e. 1 and 5 mg/kg body weight) beta-HCH concentrations in milk were elevated and signs of liver enzyme induction were found in the pups.

As significant excretion in milk was shown to occur in cows after oral dosing (the carry-over was 30-37%) (Heeschen, 1985).

6.4 Metabolic transformation

6.4.1 Rat

In a study by Freal & Chadwick (1973), Sprague-Dawley weanling female rats were administered 2 mg beta-HCH/rat per day orally in peanut oil for 7 days. Since beta-HCH was metabolized to 2,4,6-trichlorophenol but to no other chlorophenols, it appears that *cis*-dehydrochlorination may lead exclusively to this metabolite. This study also indicated that pre-treatment with beta-HCH alters the metabolism of lindane in rats.

Rats fed 1.5 mg ^{14}C-labelled beta-HCH/kg diet for 7 days excreted 70% of the dose during these 7 days and the following 28 days. One third of the eliminated radiolabel was found in the urine. There was no unchanged beta-HCH in urine; the major urinary metabolite was 2,4,6-trichlorophenol and small amounts of trichlorohydroxymethoxybenzene, a dichlorophenol, and a trace of a tetrachlorocyclohexane isomer were found. In faeces, only 2,4,6-trichlorophenol was identified (Lay et al., 1981).

Artigas et al. (1988) applied a new method of gas chromatography-mass spectrometry (GC-MS) to identify several lindane metabolites (tetra-, penta-, and hexachlorocyclohexenes, and tetra- and pentachlorobenzene) in rat brain homogenates. Male Wistar rats were administered orally 30 mg beta-HCH/kg and were sacrificed 5 h later. The cerebella of the animals were analysed and 3.6/4.5-PCCH, 3.5/4.6-PCCH, HCCH, pentachlorobenzene, HCB, and beta-HCH were found at levels below 5 µg/kg. Beta-HCH was present at a concentration of 4.2 mg/kg tissue. This study revealed that the various HCH isomers are cleared from the brain via different metabolic pathways.

6.4.2 Mouse

When ^{14}C-labelled beta-HCH was administered intraperitoneally to male mice (strain ddY, 4 weeks old) as a single dose of 32 µg, the average urinary excretion of radioactivity within 3 days was 10%. Beta-HCH seemed to be metabolized more slowly than lindane. The principal metabolite of beta-HCH in the urine was 2,4,6-trichlorophenol

(25%), but 2,4-dichlorophenol (up to 5%) was also found. These metabolites were mainly conjugated with glucuronide or sulfate (Kurihara & Nakajima, 1974; Kurihara, 1975).

6.4.3 Human

When Engst et al. (1978) analysed the urine of occupationally exposed workers (apparently to technical-grade HCH in manufacturing processes), they found, apart from alpha-, beta-, gamma-, and delta-HCH, traces of hexa- and pentachlorobenzene, gamma- and delta-pentachlorocyclohexene, pentachlorophenol, 2,3,4,5-, 2,3,4,6-, and 2,3,5,6,-tetrachlorophenol, and several trichlorophenols, as well as the glucuronides of several of these metabolites. The pentachlorocyclohexenes, tetrachlorophenol, hexachlorobenzene, and pentachlorophenol were also identified in the blood.

7. EFFECTS ON LABORATORY MAMMALS AND *IN VITRO* TEST SYSTEMS

7.1 Acute toxicity data

7.1.1 Oral

Coper et al. (1951) reported the death of three out of five rats that received a oral dose of 150 mg beta-HCH/kg body weight. Oral LD_{50} values of 1500 and 2000 mg/kg body weight for mice and rats, respectively, have been reported (WHO, 1986). However, a more recent study reported the LD_{50} to be > 16 000 mg/kg body weight in mice and > 8000 mg/kg body weight in rats (Hoffmann, 1983). Symptoms of poisoning were decreased activity, ataxia, tremors, dyspnoea, anorexia, convulsions, and rough fur. Portig (1983) reported a rat LD_{50} of 9000 mg/kg body weight.

7.1.2 Intraperitoneal

In a study by Coper et al. (1951), no deaths occurred among 6 rats given an intraperitoneal dose of 160 mg beta-HCH/kg body weight.

7.2 Short-term exposure

7.2.1 Mouse oral studies

Groups of 10-11 DD mice of each sex (6 weeks of age) received diets containing 0, 100, 300, or 600 mg beta-HCH per kg diet for 32 weeks, followed by a control diet for 5-6 weeks. The control group consisted of 20 animals. During the experiment a number of animals died. The frequency of atypical proliferation in the liver was 0/29 in the control group, 0/18 at 100 mg/kg, 6/16 at 300 mg/kg, and 11/12 at 600 mg/kg. No tumours were found (Hanada et al., 1973).

Ito et al. (1973b) fed DD mice 0, 50, 100, 200, or 500 mg beta-HCH/kg diet for 24 weeks but found no liver tumours or nodular hyperplasia.

7.2.2 Rat oral studies

In a study by Doisy & Bocklage (1950), all rats (20 weanling male) administered 0.6 g beta-HCH/kg diet for 4 weeks died within 3 weeks.

Rats administered beta-HCH at a dietary concentration of 600 mg/kg were reported to undergo growth retardation, liver mass enlargement, and a decrease in absolute brain mass, beta-HCH residues being found primarily in the fat and adrenals (Macholz et al., 1986).

A 13-week oral toxicity study with beta-HCH (> 98%) in SPF-derived Wistar RIV:Tox rats (10 male and 10 female per group) has been carried out. The levels were 0 (< 0.01), 2, 10, 50, or 250 mg/kg diet, clinical signs, growth, food intake, and organ weights were checked, and biochemical, haematological, and extensive histopathological investigations were carried out. At the highest concentration, half of the animals died following ataxia, progressive inactivity, and coma. Growth inhibition was only observed in this concentration, and red and white blood cell concentrations were decreased. The liver glycogen level was significantly higher in the group fed 250 mg/kg than in control rats. Furthermore, a significantly higher activity of aniline hydroxylase (AH) and aminopyrin-N-demethylase (APDM) microsomal enzymes and a higher concentration of cytochrome P450 were observed. In the group fed 50 mg/kg only APDM activity was increased. In all groups of treated rats, liver effects were observed (increase in organ weight, centrilobular hepatocytic hypertrophy, and proliferation of smooth endoplasmic reticulum or increased activity of microsomal enzymes). The thymus weight was significantly decreased at 50 and 250 mg/kg and the testes weight at 250 mg. At 2 mg/kg the only effect found was liver enzyme induction (van Velsen, 1986; van Velsen et al., 1986).

When young male Wistar rats were administered 800 mg beta-HCH/kg diet for 2 weeks, liver weight was increased but no differences in the content of water, nitrogen, protein, or glycogen were found. Liver fat content was increased and the DNA content per kg tissue was decreased, but the whole liver DNA content was increased. The most predominant change in the liver was hypertrophy of the liver cells. The testes weight was not different from that of the control animals but the protein content was higher. The testicular DNA content was lower than in control animals. The histological changes reported were testicular tubular atrophy, interstitial oedema, and spermatogenic arrest (Srinivasan et al., 1988).

In a study by Srinivasan et al. (1984), eight young male Wistar rats were fed 800 mg beta-HCH/kg diet for two weeks, and a control group of five rats was used. Special attention was given to the urinary excretion of body constituents reflecting renal function. Glucosuria, increased excretion of creatinine and urea, and hypertrophy and degeneration of the renal tubular epithelia were observed.

In another study with male Wistar rats fed 0 or 800 mg beta-HCH/kg diet for two weeks, special attention was given to liver function. The control group consisted of 8 rats and the treated group of 12 animals. The HCH isomer produced effects on various enzyme systems: serum aminotransferase, hepatic glucose-6-phosphate dehydrogenase, and aldolase activities were increased, while liver glucose-6-phosphatase activity was decreased. The activities of liver mitochondrial $DNP/Mg^{2+}/Ca^{2+}$-activated ATPase and liver microsomal Na^+/K^+-ATPase were lower in the treated animals (Srinivasan & Radhakrishnamurty, 1988).

Two 13-week feeding studies (Loeber & van Velsen, 1985; van Velsen et al., 1986) showed similar atrophy of the testes, with reduced tubular area, lack of mature spermatozoa, and oedema of the interstitial spaces. In both studies, only the highest beta-HCH concentration (150 mg/kg diet in one study and 250 mg/kg diet in the other) produced these effects and resulted in a significantly reduced weight gain in the affected animals. The measurement of circulating hormone levels (testosterone, FSH, LH) showed no dose-related effects. No clear endocrine effects on the testes or on male reproductive hormones were demonstrated (van Velsen, 1986).

7.3 Skin and eye irritation; sensitization

No data are available on skin and eye irritation or sensitization.

7.4 Long-term exposure

7.4.1 Rat oral studies

In a study by Fitzhugh et al. (1950), groups of 10 female and 10 male weanling Wistar rats were administered diets containing 0, 10, 100, or 800 mg beta-HCH/kg (in corn oil) for 107 weeks. With concentrations of 100 mg/kg diet or more, there was growth depression, and with 800 mg/kg increased mortality was found. Concentrations of 10 mg/kg or more led to liver enlargement and slight or moderate histopathological changes in the liver.

7.5 Reproduction, embryotoxicity, and teratogenicity

7.5.1 Reproduction

A 2-generation study with SPF-derived Wistar RIV:Tox rats (13 males and 26 females per group) was carried out to study fertility, reproduction, and development of the offspring. The parents (F_0) were fed beta-HCH (> 98%) from weaning at levels of 0 (< 0.01), 2, 10, or 50 mg/kg, and, following a 12-week premating period, F_{1a} and F_{1b} litters were produced. The F_{1b} generation was used to produce F_{2a}, F_{2b}, and F_{2c} litters, the last-mentioned being used for teratological investigations (see section 7.5.2). In the highest-dose group, the F_{1a} litter size was reduced and there was almost complete infertility when mating for the F_{1b} generation took place. All pups in this group died before weaning. At a concentration of 10 mg/kg diet, increased mortality in F_{1a} and F_{1b} litters was observed. In this group, precocious vaginal opening and complete infertility in the second generation were observed. There were no effects in the 2-mg/kg group (van Velsen, 1986).

The parental animals (F_0) from the above study were used to investigate the influence of beta-HCH on the endocrine organs after 40 weeks of exposure. In females, mean autopsy body weight and ovary weight were decreased, but adrenal gland and uterus weight increased. The organ weight changes in males were less clear, except for an increase in the weight of pituitary and adrenal glands. The proportion of animals without corpora lutea in the ovaries was greater in the group fed 50 mg/kg than it was in control rats. The testes in the animals fed at this level showed a reduced number of Leydig cells. Atrophy of the dorsolateral prostate, seminal vesicles, and coagulation glands was found in one animal. The pituitary glands of the treated animals revealed no differences in the immunoreactivity for prolactin. The pregnancy index (number of females with litters/number of females mated) was less than 0.5 in all groups of rats. Normally this strain produced pregnancy indices of nearly 1.0. The study was performed using a semi-synthetic purified feed as compared to the conventional feed used in the breeding colony. The age of females at first delivery was 20 weeks, much higher than normal. These factors cast some doubt on the results (van Velsen, 1986).

7.5.2 Teratogenicity

The F_{2c} litter from the study described in 7.5.1 was used to investigate the teratogenic effects of beta-HCH. The females were killed 20 days following sperm detection or 20 days after the last mating of the F_{1b} generation, and fetuses were inspected for internal and skeletal abnormalities. No compound-related increase in teratogenic effects was found (van Velsen, 1986).

7.6 Mutagenicity and related end-points

The available data are limited. Beta-HCH did not induce mutations in *Salmonella typhimurium* strains TA98, TA100, TA1535, or TA1537 (Lawlor & Haworth, 1979; Nishimura, 1982). The result of an *in vivo* bone marrow metaphase analysis in rats was reported to be positive (Shimazu et al., 1976; IARC, 1979). Beta-HCH did not induce mutations in *Allium cepa* roots (Nybom & Knutsson, 1947).

A mutagen test strain of *Bacillus subtilis* (TKJ5211) showed a higher sensitivity for his$^+$ reversion than the parental strain (HA101) when treated with UV and UV-mimetic chemicals. However, a negative result was obtained at a level of beta-HCH (dissolved in DMSO) of 5 mg/ml (Tanooka, 1977).

In a repair test using stationary phase cultures of HLL3g and HJ-15 strains, in which the size of growth inhibition zones of repair-proficient and repair-deficient cells (for vegetative cells and spores) was determined, a level of 5 mg beta-HCH (in benzene) per ml was without effect (Tanooka, 1977).

A thorough evaluation of the mutagenic potency of beta-HCH requires additional tests.

7.7 Carcinogenicity

Appraisal

In one study on mice, a beta-HCH dose exceeding the MTD produced an increased incidence of benign and malignant liver tumours. All other reported studies on mice were inadequate for the evaluation of beta-HCH carcinogenicity due to the very short duration of treatment and/or observation.

Two studies on rats were inadequate for evaluation due to the small number of animals in one and the short duration of treatment in the other.

The results of the studies on initiation-promotion and mode of action and the mutagenicity studies suggest that the neoplastic response observed with beta-HCH is most likely due to a non-genotoxic mechanism.

7.7.1 Mouse

In a study by Goto et al. (1972a), 20 male ICR/JCL mice (5-week old) were fed 0 or 600 mg beta-HCH/kg diet for 26 weeks. Increased liver weights were reported and hepatomas described as benign liver tumours were induced. However, insufficient details were reported.

Nagasaki (1973) administered beta-HCH orally to male DD mice at concentrations of 100, 250, or 500 mg/kg for 24 weeks. There were no signs of tumour development at any treatment level.

Groups of 10-11 DD mice of both sexes (6-weeks old) received diets containing 0, 100, 300, or 600 mg beta-HCH per kg for 32 weeks, followed by a control diet for 5-6 weeks. The control group consisted of 20 animals. During the experiment a number of animals died. In the treated mice, atypical proliferation was found in the liver in the two highest dose levels, but no hepatomas were observed. Alpha-fetoprotein was not detected in the serum of animals with hepatomas (Hanada et al., 1973).

Thorpe & Walker (1973) performed a 110-week study, using a dietary concentration of 200 mg beta-HCH (> 99%) per kg, on CF1 mice (groups of 30 males and 30 females). During the first 3 months of the study 12% of the males and 25% of the females died. Liver enlargement was detected by week 50 in both females and males. Hyperplastic changes were found in the liver (hyperplastic nodules and hepatocellular carcinomas), sometimes with lung metastases. The combined incidence of benign and malignant liver tumours for males and females was 24 and 23%, respectively, in the control group and 73 and 43%, respectively, in the treated group.

When male DD mice (8 weeks old), in groups of 20 or 29 animals, were fed a diet containing 0, 100, 250, or 500 mg beta-HCH per kg for 24 weeks, there was a moderate increase in liver weight at the two highest levels. No nodules classified as nodular hyperplasia or hepatocellular carcinoma were detected (Ito et al., 1973b).

7.7.2 Rat

In a study by Fitzhugh et al. (1950), groups of 10 male and 10 female weanling Wistar rats were fed throughout their lives on a diet containing beta-HCH > 98% pure (10, 100, or 800 mg/kg diet). No increase in tumour incidence was reported in the treated animals, but only a limited number of organs were examined microscopically.

Male W rats (5-8 weeks old, 18-24 animals per group) were administered diets containing beta-HCH at a concentration of 500 mg/kg (for 24 or 48 weeks) or 1000 mg/kg (for 24 weeks). Only slight cell hypertrophy was found, but no nodular hyperplasia, bile duct proliferation or hepatocellular carcinomas were detected (Ito et al., 1975).

7.7.3 Initiation-promotion

The influence of beta-HCH on tumour induction by PCBs (and vice versa) was tested with male DD mice (26-30 animals per group). Whereas 500 mg PCBs/kg diet induced nodular hyperplasia and hepatocellular carcinomas in the liver of male mice after 32 weeks, exposure to beta-HCH at levels of 50, 100, or 250 mg/kg diet or to PCBs at a level of 250 mg/kg diet did not. However, the combination of 100 mg beta-HCH/kg and 250 mg PCB/kg caused the induction of nodular hyperplasia in 17% (5/30) of the mice and hepatocellular carcinoma in 3.3% (1/30). The corresponding values for the combination of 250 mg beta-HCH/kg and 250 mg PCB/kg were 55% (16/29) and 21% (6/29), respectively. These results showed that PCBs promoted the hepatocarcinogenic action of beta-HCH (Ito et al., 1973a).

The tumour-initiating activity of beta-HCH has been studied by examining for phenotypically altered foci in female Wistar rats. Groups of three to eight rats were used and, after the median and right liver lobes had been removed, the rats were administered 100 mg beta-HCH/kg body weight followed by phenobarbital at 50 mg/kg body weight per day for 15 weeks. Liver foci were identified by means of the gamma-glutamyltransferase (GGT) reaction and by morphological alterations. No evidence of initiating activity was found. In another part of the study, the promoting activity was investigated. A single dose of N-nitrosomorpholine (250 mg/kg body weight by gavage) was followed by the administration of beta-HCH (0.03, 0.2, 1.0, 3.0, or 10.0 mg/kg body weight per day) for 4, 15, and 20 weeks. The criteria used were growth and phenotypic changes of foci as end-points. It was concluded from the study that beta-HCH is a tumour promotor. Both the number and size of altered foci were enhanced by a beta-HCH dose of 3 mg/kg. The tumour-promoting action was generally associated with liver growth and induction of monooxygenases or other specific enzymes (Schröter et al., 1987).

7.7.4 Mode of action

Sagelsdorff et al. (1983) studied the relevance to the carcinogenic action of HCH isomers of covalent binding to mouse liver DNA. NMRI mice were given 7.3-7.7 mg beta-HCH per kg body weight orally and ^{14}C-thymidine intraperitoneally. A very low covalent binding index (CBI) of < 0.08 was found.

7.8 Special studies

7.8.1 Effects on endocrine organs

Juvenile female Swiss mice and SPF-derived Wistar rats (RIV:Tox) were used to study the uterotropic effect of beta-HCH, in comparison with that of 17-alpha-ethynylestradiol, using the method of Tiecco (1961). Beta-HCH levels of up to 500 mg/kg diet were fed for 5 days, and in both animal species there were clear uterotropic effects at 50 mg/kg or more. In quantitative terms, the estrogenic potency of beta-HCH was, however, minimal in comparison to that of 17-alpha-ethynylestradiol (Loeber & van Velsen, 1985).

Other parameters of estrogenic potency have also been studied. Beta-HCH has been shown to increase the uterine concentration of progesterone receptors and the immunoreactivity of the adenohypophysis for prolactin in rats, and to cause the redistribution of human tumour cell receptors for progesterone. Adrenalectomy and ovariectomy did not counteract the uterotropic effect of beta-HCH in rats. However, the principal metabolite of beta-HCH, 2,4,6-trichlorophenol, had no estrogenic effect, and beta-HCH did not displace 17-beta-estradiol from its receptors (van Velsen, 1986). Both the significance of these observations and the possible mechanisms of action are unclear.

7.8.2 Neurotoxicity

Beta-HCH may raise the threshold for electrically induced seizures in rats. The ratio of the beta-HCH concentration in the brain to that in blood indicates that this isomer passes the blood-brain barrier less readily than the other HCH isomers.

Vohland et al. (1981) studied the neuropharmacological effects of beta-HCH in Wistar rats. The kinetics of beta-HCH concentrations in the brain were established after the administration of a single oral dose of 200 mg/kg body weight. The approximate half-life for elimination from the brain was 20 days in females. Beta-HCH did not give rise to appreciable quantities of hydrophobic metabolites in the brain. In rats 4-5 mg beta-HCH/kg in the brain had an anti-convulsive effect (i.e. there was protection against the action of pentylene tetrazole). Neurotoxic effects (ataxia and adynamia) occurred at brain levels of 15-20 mg beta-HCH/kg (Vohland et al., 1981; Portig & Vohland, 1983).

Beta-HCH has been demonstrated to cause a decrease in peripheral nerve conduction velocity in rats fed 600 mg beta-HCH/kg diet for 30 days, but did not cause a change in the fronto-occipital electroencephalogram at 3000 mg/kg diet (Müller et al. 1981). A decrease in absolute brain mass was reported in one study in which rats were fed beta-HCH for 30 days at a dietary concentration of 600 mg/kg (Macholz et al. 1986). Beta-HCH has been reported to raise the seizure threshold for pentylenetetrazol, a known convulsant (Vohland et al., 1981; Portig & Vohland, 1983). It has been shown that beta-HCH blocks the binding of *tert*-butylbicyclophosphorothionate (TBPS), a ligand known to bind to the GABA receptors in chloride channels in the brain, but was the least effective of the various HCH isomers in this respect (Fishman, 1987; Matsumoto et al., 1988).

7.8.3 Effect on liver enzymes

Several short-term studies on enzyme induction have been performed in rats, using levels ranging from 0.4 to 800 mg/kg feed. The highest dose level without effect in one study was 10 mg/kg body weight (van Hoof et al., 1982). However, in other studies, in which the same parameters were determined, the levels without effects included 50 mg/kg body weight. Histopathological changes in the liver correlated with the induction of microsomal enzymes (den Tonkelaar et al., 1981; van Hoof et al., 1982; van Giersbergen et al., 1984).

Weanling male rats fed diets of 800 mg beta-HCH/kg for 14-18 days showed significant increases in hepatic alanine aminotransferase (80%) and glucose-6-phosphate dehydrogenase (130%) and statistically significant decreases in hepatic aspartate aminotransferase (130%), alkaline phosphatase (45%), and acid phosphatase (40%) (Srinivasan & Radhakrishnamurty, 1977). Similarly, the dietary administration of 800 mg/kg to albino rats for two weeks resulted in noticeable hepatocellular damage, as indicated by elevations in the activity of serum aminotransferases and decreases in that of hepatic soluble enzymes. An increase in glucose-6-phosphate dehydrogenase and aldolase activities was reported to suggest a higher rate of glucose oxidation, while a decrease in liver glucose-6-phosphatase activity was attributed to an inactivation of hepatic gluconeogenesis (Srinivasan & Radhakrishnamurty, 1988).

7.8.4 Immunosuppression

To investigate potential effects on the reproductive and immune systems, beta-HCH (0, 100, or 300 mg/kg diet) was fed to groups of six female $B6C3F_1$ mice for 30 days. Investigations were conducted on changes in ovarian and uterine histology, body weight, lymphoid organ weight and histology, splenic cellularity, antigen-specific IgM and IgG plaque-forming cells (PFC), proliferative responses to mitogens, natural killer cell activity, and induction of cytosolic T lymphocytes. Significant changes in several immune functions were only found at a beta-HCH concentration of 300 mg/kg. The proliferation of splenocytes to the mitogens lipopolysaccharide (LPS), phytohaemagglutinin (PHA), and concanavalin A and T-lymphocyte-mediated cytolysis of tumour targets were decreased, and a concurrent reduction in natural killer activity was found. These data indicate that beta-HCH causes non-estrogenic immune function changes without significant changes in lymphoid organ weight, histology or cellularity (Cornacoff et al., 1988).

8. EFFECTS ON HUMANS

8.1 Acute toxicity - poisoning incidents

Several cases of acute poisoning by technical-grade HCH, resulting either from accident or occupational exposure have been described (WHO, 1991). It is likely that gamma-HCH, the most acutely toxic component, played the major role in these incidents. These cases cannot, therefore, assist in the evaluation of beta-HCH.

8.2 General population

No specific studies relating to beta-HCH are available.

A study comparing liver cancer deaths in the USA and the "domestic disappearance" of organochlorine pesticides revealed that in 1962, 18 and 15 years after the introduction of DDT and technical-grade HCH, respectively (when an increase in primary liver cancer due to the organochlorines would be manifest), the number of cases of primary liver cancer as a percentage of the total number of liver cancer deaths began a gradual and steady decline (from 61.3% in 1962 to 56.9% in 1972). The death rate (per 100 000 per year) due to primary liver cancer declined from 3.46 to 3.18 during this period (Deichmann & MacDonald, 1977).

8.3 Occupational exposure

The evaluation of the effects of beta-HCH on occupationally exposed workers is seriously hampered by the fact that most of the relevant studies relate to workers who were exposed during the manufacture and handling of lindane, or the handling and spraying of technical-grade HCH among other pesticides, and were thus exposed to all HCH isomers plus impurities and other (process) chemicals. Therefore, it is difficult, if not impossible, to relate the observed effects to individual substances. Consequently these studies have only been described in this monograph where they aid the evaluation.

Behrbohm & Brandt (1959) described 26 cases of allergic and toxic dermatitis that arose during the manufacture of technical-grade HCH. Patch testing with pure alpha-, beta-, gamma-, and delta-HCH yielded negative results, but positive reactions were obtained with the residual fractions.

The level of beta-HCH was determined in the serum of 57 workers at a lindane-manufacturing plant. No beta-HCH was detected in controls, but the levels in exposed workers ranged from 17 to 760 µg/litre and increased with the duration of exposure. The beta-HCH levels found in the adipose tissue of eight of these workers was 18-103 mg/kg (in extractable lipids). There were no clinical signs or symptoms and no significant changes were found in extensive biochemical, haematological, and neurophysiological tests, or in the EMG or EEG. Serum leutinizing hormone levels were higher than in the controls, but FSH and testosterone levels showed only insignificant and inconclusive changes (Baumann et al., 1980, 1981; Brassow et al., 1981; Tomczak et al., 1981).

The serum beta-HCH level of malaria-control workers who sprayed technical-grade HCH for 16 weeks increased from 58 to 250 µg/litre in previously non-exposed workers and from 294 to 385 µg/litre in those that had been exposed during three previous spraying seasons (Gupta et al., 1982). Although beta-HCH is only a minor component of technical-grade HCH (7-10%), it reached higher levels and persisted longer in the serum than either alpha- or gamma-HCH.

Nigam et al. (1986) studied 64 employees from a HCH-manufacturing plant who were directly or indirectly associated with the production of this insecticide. The exposed group was composed of 19 "handlers" (who handled and packed the insecticide), 26 "non-handlers" (plant operators and supervisors exposed indirectly to HCH), and 19 maintenance staff (who visited the plant frequently). The control group consisted of 14 workers who had no occupational contact with the insecticide. The exposure period varied up to 30 years. The mean serum beta-HCH concentrations in the four groups were 28.5 µg/litre (controls), 97.2 µg/litre (maintenance staff), 206.7 µg per litre (non-handlers), and 413.1 µg/litre (handlers). Alpha-, gamma-, and delta-HCH were also present. The total HCH concentrations were 51.4, 143.6, 265.6, and

604 µg/litre, respectively. Clinical examination revealed that the majority of the workers from the "handler" and "non-handler" groups exhibited paraesthesia of the face and extremities, headache, and giddiness, and some of them also showed symptoms of malaise, vomiting, tremors, apprehension, confusion, loss of sleep, impaired memory, and loss of libido. The same symptoms were found among the maintenance staff but were less severe and less frequent.

Chattopadhyay et al. (1988) studied 45 male workers exposed to HCH during its manufacture and compared them with 22 matched controls. Exposure was mainly via the skin. Paraesthesia of face and extremities, headache, giddiness, vomiting, apprehension, and loss of sleep, as well as some changes in liver function tests, were reported and were found to be related more to the intensity of exposure (as measured by the HCH levels in blood serum) than to the duration of exposure. The measured exposures to total HCH were 13 to 20 times higher than those in the control groups (no detailed figures were reported). Of the total HCH, 60-80% was beta-HCH.

Fitzhugh et al. (1950) drew attention to the importance of beta-HCH for the long-term toxicity of HCH. The slower metabolism of the beta isomer and its consequent longer persistence in the body are significant factors.

A significant correlation between the beta-HCH levels in human blood and adipose tissue has been described by Radomski et al. (1971a) and Baumann et al. (1980).

In a group of workers that were no longer exposed to HCH for at least 5 years, mean beta-HCH levels of 50 µg/litre were found, i.e. twice as much as in the general population of that area at that time (Radomski et al., 1971b).

Similar findings were reported by Morgan & Lin (1978), who found 20-348 µg/litre in the serum of 38 healthy workers whose last occupational exposure to HCH was 10-15 years previously. Liver function was normal and there were no indications of bone-marrow damage.

9. EFFECTS ON OTHER ORGANISMS IN THE LABORATORY AND FIELD

9.1 Algae

Palmer & Maloney (1955) used beta-HCH in a preliminary screening test with two cyanobacterium (blue alga), two green alga, and two diatom species. The test concentration was 2 mg/litre water and the incubation period was 3-21 days. Beta-HCH was not toxic at this concentration.

Zhou et al. (1986) studied the effects of alpha-, beta-, gamma-, and delta-HCH on the photosynthetic evolution of oxygen by the green algae *Chlorella vulgaris* and *Scenedesmus obliquus*, and reported that the beta- and gamma-isomers showed low toxicity, compared to the alpha- and delta-isomers, in this respect.

In a study by Krishnakumari (1977), cultures of the green alga *Scenedesmus acutus* (1, 3, or 5 days of age) were tested for sensitivity to beta-HCH at 28 °C, growth rate being used as parameter. The nominal concentrations of beta-HCH (dissolved in ethanol) were 0.5-100 mg/litre. A decrease in growth rate was observed in the 1, 3, and 5 day cultures exposed to 100, 10, and 5 mg/litre, respectively.

9.2 Protozoa

In short-term tests on *Tetrahymena*, the EC_{50} (growth) was 1.2 mg/litre (Mathur et al., 1984).

9.3 Invertebrates

In short-term tests on daphnids no effects were found at concentrations up to the limit of solubility of beta-HCH in water (about 1 mg/litre) (Janssen et al., 1987).

Canton et al. (1982) investigated long-term toxicity using *Daphnia* and obtained a no-observed-effect level (NOEL) for reproduction of 0.32 mg beta-HCH/litre.

9.4 Fish

9.4.1 Acute toxicity

In 4-day tests, beta-HCH affected the behaviour of fish. The NOEL and EC_{50} values for *Oryzias* (as well as for *Poecilia)* were 0.026 and 0.047 mg/litre, respectively (Wester et al., 1985; Wester & Canton, 1986).

In a study by Boulekbache (1980), the 48-h LC_{50} of beta-HCH (98.9%) for the guppy *(Poecilia reticulata)* was 0.9 mg/litre. Female fish were less sensitive than males.

9.4.2 Longer-term toxicity

Two tests were carried out with beta-HCH (98.9%) in Japanese ricefish (medaka, *Oryzias latipes)* using fertilized eggs (40 eggs/group) or 25 young fish (1 month after hatching). The exposure levels ranged from 0.032-1.0 mg beta-HCH/litre water and histopathological examinations were performed after 1 and 3 months. In the experiment on eggs, decreased growth was noted at 0.56 mg/litre; with young fish this occurred at 0.1 mg/litre. The NOELs for abnormal behaviour (loss of buoyancy and balance, uncoordinated movements) were 0.056 mg/litre and 0.032 mg/litre, respectively, for the two experiments. Histopathological lesions indicating an estrogenic activity were detected. Furthermore, lesions were observed in the liver (vacuolation), kidneys (glomerular hyalinosis), and thyroid (hypertrophy) (Wester & Canton, 1986).

In a study by Wester et al. (1985), groups of 35 young guppies *(Poecilia reticulata)* (3-4 weeks old) were exposed to various concentrations of beta-HCH (98.9%) ranging from 0.0032 to 1.0 mg/litre. After 1 and 3 months of exposure, toxicological and histopathological parameters were studied. The gross NOEL was 0.032 mg/litre after both 1 and 3 months. Changes in the liver (hypertrophy of rough endoplasmic reticulum) and kidneys (accumulation of hyaline droplets in epithelium) were detected. Hypertrophy of the endocardial lining cells (attributed to the accumulation of hyaline droplets within lysosomes) was also reported.

After 3 months dysvitellogenesis was noted in the females. In males the pituitary gland cells producing gonadotrophic hormone appeared to be stimulated and testicular development was retarded at 0.32 mg/litre or more. It was suggested that all the observed effects were attributable to an excessive production of the yolk precursor vitellogenin by the liver as a result of an estrogen-like activity of beta-HCH or its metabolites.

9.5 Terrestrial organisms

9.5.1 Birds

No toxic effects (e.g., effects on body weight, food consumption, growth, egg production, egg weight, shell quality, mortality) were observed in chickens fed diets containing 1-625 mg beta-HCH/kg for 12 weeks (Kan et al., 1979).

9.6 Model ecosystem studies

Sugiura et al. (1976) studied the effects of 0.01, 0.1, 1, 3, and 5 mg beta-HCH/litre on an aquatic microcosm consisting of bacteria, ciliata, rotifera, oligochaeta, green algae, and blue-green algae. The specific growth rates of protozoans and a rotifer were increased by 0.01 and 0.1 mg/litre. No effects were found on the total community respiration, although the gross primary production increased.

CONCLUSIONS AND RECOMMENDATIONS FOR PROTECTION OF HUMAN HEALTH AND THE ENVIRONMENT (ALPHA- AND BETA-HEXACHLOROCYCLOHEXANES)

1. Conclusions

The potential adverse effects of alpha- and beta-hexachlorocyclohexanes (HCHs) on humans and the environment cannot be balanced against benefits, since these isomers have no insecticidal action. Their presence in the environment is thus of serious concern. Consequently, the use of technical-grade HCH products containing high concentrations of alpha- and beta-HCH is never justified.

1.1 General population

Alpha- and beta-HCH are circulating in the environment and present in food chains. Thus there is a continuous potential for human exposure. This exposure is low and is expected to decrease slowly in the coming years. Therefore, there is no serious health concern for the general population.

1.2 Sub-populations at special risk

Alpha-HCH concentrations in breast milk are low.

The exposure of babies resulting from present beta-HCH concentrations in breast milk is a matter of concern but is no reason for not promoting the use of breast-feeding.

However, every possible effort should be made to decrease dietary and all other exposure to these isomers. Decreased dietary exposure is expected to result in decreased levels of alpha- and beta-HCH in breast milk.

1.3 Occupational exposure

As long as recommended precautions to minimize the exposure of workers involved in lindane manufacturing are observed, alpha- and beta-HCH pose no health risk to process operators.

1.4 Environmental effects

Apart from spills into the aquatic environment, there is no evidence to suggest that the presence of alpha- and beta-HCH in the environment poses a significant hazard to populations of organisms.

2. Recommendations for protection of human health and the environment

a) In order to minimize environmental pollution with alpha- and beta-HCH, lindane (> 99% gamma-HCH) must be used instead of technical-grade HCH.

b) In order to avoid environmental pollution with alpha- and beta-HCH, by-products and effluents from the manufacturing of lindane must be disposed of in an appropriate way, and contamination of natural waters and soil must be avoided.

c) Monitoring of alpha- and beta-HCH in food should continue. It is essential that a mechanism for setting internationally acceptable levels of alpha- and beta-HCH in food be initiated.

d) Monitoring of the daily intake of the general population and the levels of alpha- and beta-HCH in breast milk should continue.

FURTHER RESEARCH (ALPHA- AND BETA-HEXACHLOROCYCLOHEXANES)

The following experimental studies are needed to allow a better evaluation of the hazards of alpha- and beta-HCH:

- mutagenicity studies, especially with chromosome mutagenic end-points;

- reproduction and fetotoxicity/teratogenicity studies;

- pharmacokinetic and toxicokinetic studies;

- carcinogenicity studies;

- neurotoxicity studies;

- surveillance studies on populations at risk.

PREVIOUS EVALUATIONS BY INTERNATIONAL BODIES

The International Agency for Research on Cancer (IARC, 1987) evaluated the hexachlorocyclohexanes and concluded that for the technical grade and the alpha isomer there is sufficient evidence for carcinogenicity to animals, whereas this evidence is limited for the beta and gamma isomers. There is inadequate evidence for their carcinogenicity to human beings. The hexachlorocyclohexanes were classified in group 2B.

REFERENCES

ALBRO, P.W. & THOMAS, R. (1974) Intestinal absorption of hexachlorobenzene and hexachlorocyclohexane isomers in rats. Bull. environ. Contam. Toxicol., 12(3): 289-294.

ALTHAUS, F.R., LAWRENCE, S.D., SATTLER, G.L., LONGFELLOW, D.G., & PITOT, H.C. (1982) Chemical quantification of unscheduled DNA synthesis in cultured hepatocytes as an assay for the rapid screening of potential chemical carcinogens. Cancer Res., 42: 3010-3015.

ALTMANN, H.J., BÖHME, Chr., & UEHLEKE, H. (1980) Long-term kinetics of beta-hexachlorocyclohexane (beta-HCH) in rats and mini-pigs. Arch. Pharmacol., 31 (Suppl.): R20 (Abstract No. 78).

ANGSUBHAKORN, S., BHAMARAPRAVATI, N., ROMRUEN, K., SAHAPHONG, S., THAMAVIT, W., & MIYAMOTO, M. (1981) Further study of alpha-benzenehexachloride inhibition of aflatoxin B1 carcinogenesis in rats. Br. J. Cancer, 13: 881-883.

ANON. (1984) [1984 Nutrition report], Frankfurt am Main, German Nutrition Association (in German).

ARBEITSGEMEINSCHAFT FÜR DIE REINHALTUNG DER ELBE (1982) [Chlorinated hydrocarbons; data for the river Elbe. Report on the results of the programme for the measurement of chlorinated hydrocarbons in the section of the Elbe between Schnackenburg and the North Sea, 1980-1982], Hamburg, Study Group for Keeping the Elbe Clean, pp. 64-65, 84, 86-94 (in German).

ARBEITSGEMEINSCHAFT FÜR DIE REINHALTUNG DER ELBE (1988) [Water quality data for the Elbe from Schnackenburg to the sea. Numerical table, 1988], Hamburg, Study Group for Keeping the Elbe Clean, p. 158 (in German).

ARTIGAS, F., MARTINEZ, E., CAMON, L., GELPI, E., & RODRIGUEZ-FARRE, E. (1988) Brain metabolites of lindane and related isomers: Identification by negative ion mass spectrometry. Toxicology, 49: 57-63.

ATLAS, E. & GIAS, C.S. (1981) Global transport of organic pollutants: Ambient concentrations in the remote marine atmosphere. Science, 211: 163-165.

BACCI, E., CALAMARI, D., GAGGI, C., FANELLI, R., FOCARDI, S., & MOROSINI, M. (1986) Chlorinated hydrocarbons in lichen and moss samples from the Antarctic Peninsular. Chemosphere, 15(6): 747-754.

BAUER, U. (1972) [Concentration of insecticides, chlorinated hydrocarbons and PCB in algae.] Schr. Reihe Ver. Wasser-Boden-Lufthyg., 37: 211-219 (in German).

BAUMANN, K., ANGERER, J., HEINRICH, R., & LEHNERT, G. (1980) Occupational exposure to hexachlorocyclohexane. 1. Body burden of HCH-isomers. Int. Arch. occup. environ. Health, 47: 119-127.

BAUMANN, K., BEHLING, K., BRASSOW, H.L., & STAPEL, K. (1981) Occupational exposure to hexachlorocyclohexane. III. Neurophysiological findings and neuromuscular function in chronically exposed workers. Int. Arch. occup. environ. Health, 48: 165-172.

BEHRBOHM, P. & BRANDT, B. (1959) [Allergic and toxic dermatitis in the manufacturing and processing of hexachlorocyclohexane.] Arch. Gewerbepathol. Gewerbehyg., 17: 365-383 (in German).

BENSON, W.W., WATSON, M., & WYLLIE, J. (1973) Organochlorine residues in wild moose, Idaho-1972. Pestic. monit. J., 7: 97-99.

BERTRAM, H.P., KEMPER, F.H., & ZENZEN, C. (1980) [Occurrence of HCH isomers in man.] In: [Hexachlorocyclohexane as a harmful substance in foods. Papers from two symposia of the Senate Committee on the Testing of Residues in Foods, held on 28-29 November 1979 and 6 March 1980], Weinheim, Verlag Chemie, pp. 155-163 (in German).

BIDLEMAN, T.F. & LEONARD, R. (1982) Aerial transport of pesticides over the Northern Indian Ocean and adjacent seas. Atmos. Environ., 16: 1099-1107.

BLOK, S.M.G., GREVE, P.A., SANGSTER, B., SAVELKOUL, T.J.F., & WEGMAN, R.C.C. (1984) [Investigation of normally occurring values of a number of organochlorine pesticides and related compounds and their metabolites, of polychlorobiphenyls and of chlorophenols in the blood or plasma of healthy volunteers], Bilthoven, National Institute of Public Health and Environmental Hygiene (Report No. 638101001) (in Dutch).

BOULEKBACHE, H. (1980) Study of the toxicity of the alpha-, beta-, and gamma-isomers of hexachlorocyclohexane to fish, using the guppy as the test species, Paris, Université Paris VII, Laboratoire d'Anatomie comparée (Unpublished report).

BRASSOW, H.L., BAUMANN, K., & LEHNERT, G. (1981) Occupational exposure to hexachlorocyclohexane. II. Health conditions of chronically exposed workers. Int. Arch. occup. environ. Health, 48: 81-87.

BÜSSER, M.T. & LUTZ, W.K. (1987) Stimulation of DNA synthesis in rat and mouse liver by various tumour promoters. Carcinogenesis, 8(10): 1433-1437.

CAMON, L., MARTINEZ, E., ARTIGAS, F., SOLA, C., & RODRIGUEZ-FARRE, E. (1988) The effect of non-convulsant doses of lindane on temperature and body weight. Toxicology, 49: 389-394.

CANTON, J.H. & SLOOFF, W. (1977) The usefulness of *Lymnea stagnalis* L. as a biological indicator in toxicological bioassays (model substance α-HCH). Water Res., 11: 117-121.

CANTON, J.H., GREVE, P.A., SLOOFF, W., & VAN ESCH, G.J. (1975) Toxicity, accumulation, and elimination studies of α-hexachlorocyclohexane (α-HCH) with freshwater organisms of different trophic levels. Water Res., 9: 1163-1169.

CANTON, J.H., VAN ESCH, G.J., GREVE, P.A., & VAN HELLEMOND, A.B.A.M (1977) Accumulation and elimination of α-hexachlorocyclohexane (α-HCH) by the marine algae *Chlamydomonas* and *Dunaliella*. Water Res., 11: 111-115.

References

CANTON, J.H., WEGMAN, R.C.C., VULTO, Th.J.A., VERHOEF, C.H., & VAN ESCH, G.J. (1978) Toxicity-, accumulation-, and elimination-studies of α-hexachlorocyclohexane (α-HCH) with saltwater organisms of different trophic levels. Water Res., 12: 687-690.

CANTON, J.H., MENNES, W.C., MATHIJSSEN-SPIEKMAN, E.A.M., WEGMAN, R.C.C., HOFSTEE, A.W.M., & WESTER, P.W. (1982) [Study of the toxicity of beta-HCH for freshwater organisms], Bilthoven, National Institute of Public Health and Environmental Hygiene (Unpublished report No. 62797001) (in Dutch).

CETINKAYA, M., GABEL, B., PODBIELSKI, A., & THIEMANN, W. (1984) [On the correlation of nutrition and living habits of feeding mothers and contamination of human milk with non-volatile chlorinated organic chemicals.] Akt. Ernähr., 9(4): 157-162 (in German).

CHATTOPADHYAY, P., KARNIK, A.B., THAKORE, K.N., LAKKAD, B.C., NIGAM, S.K., & KASHYAP, S.K. (1988) Health effects among workers involved in the manufacture of hexachlorocyclohexane. J. Soc. Occup. Med., 38: 77-81.

CHESSELLS, M.J., HAWKER, D.W., CONNELL, D.W., & PAPAJCSIK, I.A. (1988) Factors influencing the distribution of lindane and isomers in soil of an agricultural environment. Chemosphere, 17(9): 1741-1749.

COPER, H., HERKEN, H., & KLEMPAU, I. (1951) [Antagonism and synergism of β- and γ-hexachlorocyclohexanes.] Klin. Wochenschr., 29(13/14): 264-265 (in German).

CORNACOFF, J.B., LAUER, L.D., HOUSE, R.V., TUCKER, A.N., THURMOND, L.M., VOS, J.G., WORKING, P.K., & DEAN, J.H. (1988) Evaluation of the immunotoxicity of β-Hexachlorocyclohexane (β-HCH). Fundam. appl. Toxicol., 11: 293-299.

COWAN, A.A. (1981) Organochlorine compounds in mussels from Scottish coastal waters. Environ. Pollut., B2: 129-143.

DAVIES, D. & MES, J. (1987) Comparison of the residue levels of some organochlorine compounds in breastmilk of the general and indigenous Canadian populations. Bull. environ. Contam. Toxicol., 39: 743-749.

DEICHMANN, W.B. & MACDONALD, W.E. (1977) Organochlorine pesticides and liver cancer deaths in the United States, 1930-1972. Ecotoxicol. environ. Saf., 1: 89-110.

DEMOZAY, D. & MARECHAL, G. (1972) Physical and chemical properties. In: Ulman, E., ed. Lindane: Monograph of an insecticide, Freiburg im Breisgau, Verlag K. Schillinger, pp. 14-21.

DEN TONKELAAR, E.M., VAN NIMWEGEN, J.M., & SEKHUIS, V.M. (1981) [Induction of microsomal liver enzymes following subacute administration of alpha-, beta-, and gamma-HCH to the rat], Bilthoven, National Institute of Public Health and Environmental Hygiene (Unpublished report No. 618111001) (in Dutch).

DEO, P.G., HASAN, S.B., & MAJUMDER, S.K. (1980) Isomerization of β-HCH in aqueous solution. J. environ. Sci. Health, B15(2): 147-164.

DEO, P.G., HASAN, S.B., & MAJUMDER, S.K. (1981) Interconversions and toxicity changes in hexachlorocyclohexane isomers on dispersion in water. J. environ. Sci. Health, **B16**(6): 691-701.

DFG (1978) [Residues in breast milk: situation and assessment], Boppard, Germany, Harald Boldt Verlag (in German).

DOELMAN, P., HAANSTRA, L., DE RUITER, E., & SLANGE, J., (1985) Rate of microbial degradation of high concentrations of δ-hexachlorocyclohexane in soil under aerobic and anaerobic conditions. Chemosphere, **14**(5): 565-570.

DOELMAN, P., HAANSTRA, L., & VOS, A. (1988a) Microbial degradation by the autochthonous soil population of alpha and beta-HCH under anaerobic field conditions in temperate regions. Chemosphere, **17**(2): 481-487.

DOELMAN, P., HAANSTRA, L., & VOS, A. (1988b) Microbial sanitation of soil with alpha- and beta-HCH under aerobic glass house conditions. Chemosphere, **17**(2): 489-492.

DOISY, E.A., Jr & BOCKLAGE, B.C. (1950) Inositol and the toxicity of four isomers of benzenehexachloride for the rat. Proc. Soc. Exp. Biol. Med., **74**: 613-616.

ECKENHAUSEN, F.W., BENNETT, D., BEYNON, K.I., & ELGAR, K.E. (1981) Organochlorine pesticide concentrations in perinatal samples from mothers and babies. Arch. environ. Health, **36**(2): 81-92.

EDELMAN, Th. (1984) [Background values of a number of anorganic and organic substances in the soil of the Netherlands; an initial reconnaissance], The Hague, State Publishing House (Soil protection, report VROM 34) (in Dutch).

EDER, G., STURM, R., & ERNST, W. (1987) Chlorinated hydrocarbons in sediments of the Elbe River and the estuary. Chemosphere, **16**(10/12): 2487-2496.

EGAN, H. & HUBBARD, A.W. (1975) Analytical surveys of food. Br. med. Bull., **31**(3): 201-208.

EICHLER, D. (1977) Experiments on the decomposition of lindane when exposed to UV-light (Unpublished report Celamerck No. 111AC-143-004, submitted to WHO by CIEL).

EICHLER, D., HEUPT, W., & PAUL, W. (1983) Comparative study on the distribution of alpha- and gamma-hexachlorocyclohexane in the rat with particular reference to the problem of isomerization. Xenobiotica, **13**(11): 639-647.

ENGST, R., MACHOLZ, R.M., & KUJAWA, M. (1978) [Metabolites of HCH-isomers in human blood.] Pharmazie, **33**(2/3): 109-111 (in German).

ERNST, W. (1977) Determination of the bioconcentration of marine organisms. A steady state approach. I. Bioconcentration data for seven chlorinated pesticides in mussels (Mytilus edulis) and their relation to solubility data. Chemosphere, **6**(11): 731-340.

References

ERNST, W. (1979) Factors affecting the evaluation of chemicals in laboratory experiments using marine organisms. Ecotoxicol. environ. Saf., 3: 90-98.

FALADYSZ, J. & SZEFER, D. (1982) Chlorinated hydrocarbons in diving ducks wintering in Gdansk Bay, Baltic Sea. Sci. total Environ., 24: 119-127.

FISHMAN, B.E. (1987) The neurotoxicity of the isomers of hexachlorocyclohexane: actions at the GABA-A-receptor linked chloride channel. Diss. Abstr. Int., B48: 3257-3258.

FISHMAN, B.E. & GIANUTSOS, G. (1987) Opposite effects of different hexachlorocyclohexane (lindane) isomers on cerebellar cyclic GMP: relation of cyclic GMP accumulation to seizure activity. Life Sci., 41: 1703-1709.

FISHMAN, B.E. & GIANUTSOS, G. (1988) CNS biochemical and pharmacological effects of the isomers of hexachlorocyclohexane (lindane) in the mouse. Toxicol. appl. Pharmacol., 93: 146-153.

FITZHUGH, O.G., NELSON, A.A., & FRAWLEY, J.P. (1950) The chronic toxicities of technical benzene hexachloride and its alpha-, beta-, and gamma-isomers. J. Pharmacol. exp. Ther., 100(1): 59-66.

FOOKEN, C. & BUTTE, W. (1987) Organochlorine pesticides and polychlorinated biphenyls in human milk during lactation. Chemosphere, 16(6): 1301-1309.

FOSTER, T.S. & SAHA, J.G. (1978) The *in vitro* metabolisation of lindane by an enzyme preparation from chicken liver. J. environ. Sci. Health, B13(1): 25-45.

FRANK, R., BRAUN, H.E., SIRONS, G.H., RASPER, J., & WARD, G.G. (1985) Organochlorine and organophosphorus insecticides and industrial pollutants in the milk supplies of Ontario, 1983. J. Food Prod., 48(6): 499-504.

FRANKLIN, A. (1987) The concentration of metals, organochlorine pesticide and PCB residues in marine fish and shell fish: results from MAFF fish and shell fish monitoring programmes, 1977-1984, Lowestoft, Ministry of Agriculture, Fisheries, and Food, Directorate of Fisheries Research (Aquatic Environment Monitoring Report No. 16).

FREAL, J.J. & CHADWICK, R.W. (1973) Metabolism of hexachlorocyclohexane to chlorophenols and effect of isomer pretreatment on lindane metabolism in rat. J. agric. food Chem., 21(3): 424-427.

GAGGI, C., BACCI, E., CALAMARI, D., & FANELLI, R. (1986) Chlorinated hydrocarbons in plant foliage: An indication of the tropospheric contamination level. Chemosphere, 14(11-12): 1673-1686.

GARTRELL, M.J., CRAUN, J.C., PODREBARAC, D.S., & GUNDERSON, E.L. (1985a) Pesticides, selected elements and other chemicals in adult total diet samples, October 1978-September 1979. J. Assoc. Off. Anal. Chem., 68(5): 862-875.

GARTRELL, M.J., CRAUN, J.C., PODREBARAC, D.S., & GUNDERSON, E.L. (1985b) Pesticides, selected elements and other chemicals in Infant and

Toddler total diet samples, October 1978-September 1979. J. Assoc. Off. Anal. Chem., 68(5): 842-861.

GEYER, H., SCHEUNERT, I., & KORTE, F. (1986) Bioconcentration potential of organic environmental chemicals in humans. Regul. Toxicol. Pharmacol., 6: 313-347.

GOTO, M., HATTORI, M., & MIYAGAWA, T. (1972a) [Contributions to ecological chemistry. II. Hepatoma formation in mice after administration of high doses of HCH isomers.] Chemosphere, 6: 279-282 (in German).

GOTO, M., HATTORI, M., & MIYAGAWA, T. (1972b) [Contributions to ecological chemistry. Toxicity of alpha-BHC in mice.] Chemosphere, 4: 153-154 (in German).

GREVE, P.A. (1985) Organochlorine pesticides and PCBs in human tissues from Dutch citizens (1968-1983), Bilthoven, National Institute of Public Health and Environmental Hygiene (Unpublished concept report).

GREVE, P.A. & VAN HARTEN, D.C. (1983) [Relationship between levels of organochlorine pesticides and PCBs in fat and blood in human subjects], Bilthoven, National Institute of Public Health and Environmental Hygiene (Unpublished report No. 638219001) (in Dutch).

GREVE, P.A. & VAN HULST, Sj. (1977) [Organochlorine pesticides and PCBs in duplicate 24-hour feeds], Bilthoven, National Institute of Public Health and Environmental Hygiene (Unpublished report No. 192/77 Tox/ROB) (in Dutch).

GREVE, P.A. & VAN HULST, Sj. (1980) [Content of beta- and gamma-HCH and some of their metabolites in rat tissues derived from the semi-chronic toxicity tests], Bilthoven, National Institute of Public Health and Environmental Hygiene (Unpublished report No. 144/80, RA/617908001) (in Dutch).

GREVE, P.A. & WEGMAN, R.C.C. (1985) Organochlorine compounds in human milk; data from a recent investigation in the Netherlands. Working paper for WHO Consultation on Organochlorine Compounds in Human Milk and Related Hazards, Bilthoven, 9-11 January, 1985, Bilthoven, National Institute of Public Health and Environmental Hygiene.

GUICHERIT, R. & SCHULTING, F.L. (1985) The occurrence of organic chemicals in the atmosphere of the Netherlands. Sci. total Environ., 43: 193-219.

GUNDERSON, E.L. (1988) FDA total diet study, April 1982-April 1984. Dietary intakes of pesticides, selected elements and other chemicals. J. Assoc. Off. Anal. Chem., 71(6): 1200-1209.

GUPTA, S.K., PARIKH, J.R., SHAH, M.P., CHATTERJEE, S.K., & KASHYAP, S.K. (1982) Changes in serum HCH residues in malaria spraymen after short-term occupational exposure. Arch. environ. Health, 37(1): 41-44.

HAIDER, K. (1979) Degradation and metabolization of lindane and other hexachlorocyclohexane isomers by anaerobic and aerobic soil microorganisms. Z. Naturforsch., 34C: 1066-1069.

References

HAMADA, M., KAWANO, E., KAWAMURA, S., & SHIRO, M. (1982) A new isomer of 1,2,3,4,5-pentachlorocyclohexane from UV-irradiation products of α-, β-, and δ-isomers of 1,2,3,4,5,6-hexachlorocyclohexane. Agric. biol. Chem., 46(1): 153-157.

HANADA, M., YUTANI, C., & MIYAJI, T. (1973) Induction of hepatoma in mice by benzene hexachloride. Gann., 64(5): 511-513.

HAPKE, H.J. & HOLLMANN, A.C. (1985) [Effects of beta-hexachlorocyclohexane on suckling rats.] Dtsch. Tierärztl. Wschr., 92(1): 125-164 (in German).

HEESCHEN, W. (1985) Studies on the carry-over of beta-hexachlorocyclohexane in the milk of cows. Kieler Milchwirtsch. Forschungsber., 37(1): 29-43.

HERITAGE, A.D. & MACRAE, I.C. (1977) Identification of intermediates formed during the degradation of hexachlorocyclohexanes by *Clostridium sphenoïdes*. Appl. environ. Microbiol., 33(6): 1295-1297.

HERITAGE, A.D. & MACRAE, I.C. (1979) Degradation of hexachlorocyclohexanes and structurally related substances by *Clostridium sphenoïdes*. Aust. J. biol. Sci., 32(4/5): 493-500.

HERRMANN, R., THOMAS, W., & HÜBNER, D. (1984) [Behaviour of organic micropollutants (PAH, PCB and BHC) and of a fecal sterol in the Husum estuary and in the adjacent North Frisian Wadden sea.] Dtsch. Gewässerkd. Mitt., 4: 101-107 (in German).

HILDEBRANDT, G., JEEP, H., HURKA, H., STUKE, T., HEITMAN, M., & BOISELLE, C. (1986) [Breast milk as a biological indicator: Study on the organic halogen burden in breast milk and foodstuffs], Berlin, Schmidt E. Verlag (Report 5/86 of the Federal Office for the Environment) (in German).

HMSO (1969) Further review of certain persistent organochlorine pesticides used in Great Britain. Report by the Advisory Committee on Pesticides and other Toxic Chemicals, London, Her Majesty's Stationery Office.

HMSO (1982) Report of the Working Party on Pesticide Residues (1977-1981): Ninth report of the Steering Group on Food Surveillance, London, Ministry of Agriculture, Fisheries, and Food, Her Majesty's Stationery Office (Food Surveillance Paper No. 9).

HMSO (1986) Report of the Working Party Pesticide on Residues (1982-1985): Sixteenth report of the Steering Group on Food Surveillance, London, Ministry of Agriculture, Fisheries, and Food, Her Majesty's Stationery Office (Food Surveillance Paper No. 16).

HMSO (1989) Report of the Working Party on Pesticide Residues (1985-1988): Twenty-fifth report of the Steering Group on Food Surveillance, London, Ministry of Agriculture, Fisheries, and Food, Her Majesty's Stationery Office (Food Surveillance Paper No. 25).

HOFFMANN, A. (1983) [Toxicity of alpha- and beta-HCH.] In: [Hexachlorocyclohexane as a harmful substance in foodstuffs. Papers from two seminars of the

Senate Committee on the Testing of Residues in Foodstuffs held on 28-29 November 1979 and 6 March 1980], Weinheim, Chemie Verlag, pp. 201-214 (in German).

HOLT, R.L., CRUSE, S., & GREER, E.S. (1986) Pesticide and polychlorinated biphenyl residues in human adipose tissue from North East Louisiana. Bull. environ. Contam. Toxicol., 36: 651-655.

HORI, S. & KASHIMOTO, T. (1974) Transfer of beta-HCH from mother to suckling mouse. Shokuhin Eiseigaku Zasshi, 15(6): 446-450.

IARC (1979) Hexachlorocyclohexane (technical HCH and lindane). In: Some halogenated hydrocarbons, Lyon, International Agency for Research on Cancer, pp. 195-239 (IARC Monographs on the Evaluation of the Carcinogenic Risk of Chemicals to Humans, Vol. 20).

IARC (1987) Hexachlorocyclohexanes (Group 2B). In: Overall evaluations of carcinogenicity: An updating of IARC Monographs Vol. 1 to 42, Lyon, International Agency for Research on Cancer (IARC Monographs on the Evaluation of Carcinogenic Risks to Humans, Suppl. 7).

ITO, N., NAGASAKI, H., ARAI, M., MAKIURA, S., SUGIHARA, S., & HIRAO, K. (1973a) Histopathologic studies on liver tumorigenesis induced in mice by technical polychlorinated biphenyls and its promoting effect on liver tumours induced by benzene hexachloride. J. Natl Cancer Inst., 51(5): 1637-1646.

ITO, N., NAGASAKI, H., ARAI, M., SUGIHARA, S., & MAKIURA, S. (1973b) Histologic and ultrastructural studies on the hepatocarcinogenicity of benzene hexachloride in mice. J. Natl Cancer Inst., 51(3): 817-826.

ITO, N., NAGASAKI, H., AOE, H., SUGIHARA, S., MIYATA, Y., ARAI, M., & SHIRAI, T. (1975) Brief Communication: Development of hepatocellular carcinomas in rats treated with benzene hexachloride. J. Natl Cancer Inst., 54(3): 801-905.

ITO, N., HANAOUCHI, M., SUGIHARA, S., SHIRAI, T., TSUDA, H., FUKUSHIMA, S., & NAGASAKI, H. (1976) Reversibility and irreversibility of liver tumours in mice induced by the α-isomer of 1,2,3,4,5,6,-hexachlorocyclohexane. Cancer Res., 36: 2227-2234.

ITO, N., TSUDA, H., HASEGAWA, R., & IMAIDA, K. (1983) Comparison of the promoting effects of various agents in induction of preneoplastic lesions in rat liver. Environ. Health Perspect., 50: 131-138.

IVERSON, F., RYAN, J.J., LIZOTTE, R., & HIERLIHY, S.L. (1984) *In vivo* and *in vitro* binding of α- and γ-hexachlorocyclohexane to mouse liver macromolecules. Toxicol. Lett., 20(3): 331-335.

JAGNOW, G., HAIDER, K., & ELLWARDT, P.Chr. (1977) Anaerobic dechlorination and degradation of hexachlorocyclohexane isomers by anaerobic and facultative anaerobic bacteria. Arch. Microbiol., 115: 285-292.

References

JANSSEN, P.J.C.M., VAN KOTEN-VERMEULEN, J.E.M., KRAJNC, E.I., CANTON, J.H., VAN GESTEL, C.A.M., VAN DER HEIJDEN, C.A., & HEIJNA-MERKENS, E. (1987) [Hexachlorocyclohexane (Basic document)], Bilthoven, National Institute of Public Health and Environmental Hygiene (Project No. 840820) (in Dutch).

KAMPE, W. (1980) [Occurrence of hexachlorocyclohexane in the soil.] In: [Hexachlorocyclohexane as a harmful substance in foodstuffs], Weinheim, Verlag Chemie, pp. 18-23 (Research report) (in German).

KAN, C.A. & JONKER-DEN ROOYEN, J.C. (1978a) Accumulation and depletion of some organochlorine pesticides in broiler breeder hens during the second laying cycle. J. agric. food Chem., 26(2): 465-470.

KAN, C.A. & JONKER-DEN ROOYEN, J.C. (1978b) Accumulation and depletion of some organochlorine pesticides in high producing laying hens. J. agric. food Chem., 26(4): 935-940.

KAN, C.A., JONKER-DEN ROOYEN, J.C., TUINSTRA, L.G.M.Th., ROOS, A.H., & TRAUG, W. (1978) Possible influence of sex and embryonic content on accumulation of some organochlorine pesticides in broilers. J. agric. food Chem., 26(3): 618-621.

KAN, C.A., STRIK, J.J.T.W.A., & KOEMAN, J.H. (1979) Semi-chronic toxicity of beta-HCH in laying hens. Meded. Fac. Landbouwwet. Rijksuniv. Gent, 44(2): 965-973.

KORANSKY, W., PORTIG, J., & MÜNCH, G. (1963) [Absorption, distribution and excretion of α- and γ-hexachlorocyclohexane.] Naunyn-Schmiedebergs Arch. exp. Pathol. Pharmakol. 244: 564-575 (in German).

KORANSKY, W., PORTIG, J., VOHLAND, H.W., & KLEMPAU, I. (1964) [Elimination of α- and γ-hexachlorocyclohexane and the way it is influenced by enzymes of liver microsomes.] Naunyn-Schmiedebergs Arch. exp. Pathol. Pharmakol., 247: 49-60 (in German).

KORTE, F. (1980) [Occurrence of HCH isomers in man.] In: [Hexachlorocyclohexane as a harmful substance in foodstuffs. Papers from two seminars of the Senate Committee on the Testing of Residues in Foodstuffs held on 28-29 November 1979 and 6 March 1980], Weinheim, Verlag Chemie, pp. 46-64 (in German).

KRAUS, D. (1975) Biodegradation of alpha-hexachlorocyclohexane by microsomes and cytosol of rat liver. Naunyn-Schmiedebergs Arch. Pharmakol., 291: 79-87.

KRAUTHACKER, B., ALEBIC-KOLBAH, T., KRALJ, M., TKALCEVIC, B., & REINER, E. (1980) Organochlorine pesticides in blood serum of the general Yugoslav population and in occupationally exposed workers. Int. Arch. occup. environ. Health, 45: 217-220.

KRISHNAKUMARI, M.K. (1977) Sensitivity of the alga *Scenedesmus acutus* to some pesticides. Life Sci., 20: 1525-1532.

KUIPER, H.A., DEN TONKELAAR, E.M., VAN LEEUWEN, F.X.R., FRANKEN, M.A.M., & DORMANS, J.A.M.A. (1985) [Semi-chronic toxicity test with alpha-

HCH], Bilthoven, National Institute of Public Health and Environmental Hygiene (Report No. 617917002) (in Dutch).

KURIHARA, N. (1975) Urinary metabolites from β- and γ-HCH in the mouse: chlorophenol conjugates. Environ. Qual. Saf., 4: 56-73.

KURIHARA, N. & NAKAJIMA, M. (1974) Studies on BHC isomers and related compounds VIII. Urinary metabolites produced from γ- and β-BHC in the mouse: Chlorophenol conjugates. Pestic. Biochem. Physiol., 4: 220-231.

KUTZ, F.W., STRASSMAN, S.C., & SPERLING, J.F. (1979) Survey of selected organochlorine pesticides in the general population of the United States: Fiscal years 1970-1975. Ann. NY Acad. Sci., 320: 60-68.

LAUGEL, P. (1981) [The residue situation in France and ways of overcoming it.] Lebensmittelchem. gerichtl. Chem., 35: 29-32 (in German).

LAWLOR, T. & HAWORTH, S.R. (1979) Evaluation of the genetic activity of nine chlorinated phenols, seven chlorinated benzenes and three chlorinated hexanes. Environ. Mutagen., 1(2): 143.

LAY, J.P., KLEIN, W., KORTE, F., & RICHTER, E. (1981) Metabolism of β-hexachlorocyclohexane-[^{14}]C in rats following low dosing in the daily diet. J. environ. Sci. Health, B16: 227- 238.

LOEBER, J.G. & VAN VELSEN, F.L. (1985) Uterotropic effect of β-HCH. A food chain contaminant. Food Addit. Contam., 1: 63-66.

LOWDEN, G.F., SAUNDERS, C.L., & EDWARDS, R.W. (1969) Organochlorine insecticides in water (Part II). J. Water Treat. Exam., 18: 275-287.

LWA (1987) [Water quality report], Düsseldorf, North-Rhine Westphalia Office for Water and Refuse, 24 pp (in German).

MACHOLZ, R.M., KNOLL, R., LEWERENZ, H.J., PETRZIKA, M., & ENGST, R. (1982) Metabolism of alpha-hexachlorocyclohexane. Free metabolites in urine and organs of rats. Xenobiotica, 12(4): 227-231.

MACHOLZ, R.M., KNOLL, R., LEWERENZ, H.J., PLASS, R., & SCHULZE, J. (1983) [Metabolism of gamma-hexachlorocyclohexane (HCH) in germ-free and conventionalized rats.] Zentralbl. Pharm., 122(2): 221 (in German).

MACHOLZ, R.M., BLEYL, D.W., KLEPEL, H., KNOLL, R., KUJAWA, M., LEWERENZ, H.J., MUELLER, D., & PLASS, R. (1986) Comparison of distribution and toxicity of alpha-, beta-, and gamma-BHC after application to rats for 30 days. Nahrung, 30: 701-708.

MACRAE, I.C., RAGHU, K., & CASTRO, T.F. (1967) Persistence and biodegradation of four common isomers of benzenehexachloride in submerged soils. J. agric. food Chem., 15(5): 911-914.

MACRAE, J.C., YAMAYA, Y., & YOSHIDA, T. (1984) Persistence of HCH-isomers in soil suspensions. Soil Biol. Biochem., 16: 285-286.

References

MARTIN, D.B. & HARTMANN, W.A. (1985) Organochlorine pesticides and polychlorinated biphenyls in sediment and fish from wetlands in the North-Central United States. J. Assoc. Off. Anal. Chem., **69**(4): 712-717.

MATHUR, R., SAXENA, D.M., & AGARWAL, H.C. (1984) Growth of a ciliate protozoan. Tetrahymena pyriformis in the presence of different isomers of hexachlorocyclohexane (HCH). Acta. Protozool., **23**(3): 165-174.

MATSUMOTO, K., ELDERFRAWI, M.E., & ELDEFRAWI, A.T. (1988) Action of polychlorocycloalkane insecticides in binding of [355] t-butyldicyclophosphorothionate to torpedo electric organ membranes and stereospecificity of the binding site. Toxicol. appl. Pharmacol., **95**: 220-229.

MATSUSHIMA, S. (1972) [Pollution of food by agricultural chemicals and the diet.] Rinsho. Eiyo., **40**: 555-563 (in Japanese).

MES, J., DAVIES, D.J., & TURTON, D. (1982) Polychlorinated biphenyl and other chlorinated hydrocarbon residues in adipose tissue of Canadians. Bull. environ. Contam. Toxicol., **28**: 97-104.

MES, J., DAVIES, D.J., TURTON, D., & SUN, W.-F. (1986) Levels and trends of chlorinated hydrocarbon contaminants in the breast milk of Canadian women. Food Addit. Contam., **3**(4): 313-322.

MESTRES, R. (1974) Report of a group of experts on the content of organohalogen compounds detected between 1968 and 1972 in water, air and foodstuffs and the methods of analysis used in the nine Member States of the European Communities. Presented at the European Colloquium on Problems raised by the Contamination of Man and his Environment by Persistent Pesticides and Organohalogenated Compounds, Luxembourg, 14-16 May, 1974, Luxembourg, Commission of the European Communities (Paper No. 1).

MORGAN, D.P. & LIN, L.I. (1978) Blood-organochlorine pesticide concentrations, clinical hematology and biochemistry in workers occupationally exposed to pesticides. Arch. environ. Contam. Toxicol., **7**: 423-447.

MOUVET, C., GALOUX, M., & BERNES, A. (1985) Monitoring of polychlorinated biphenyls (PCBs) and hexachlorocyclohexanes (HCH) in freshwater using the aquatic moss *Cinclidotus danubicus*. Sci. total Environ., **44**: 253-267.

MÜLLER, D., KLEPEL, H., MACHOLZ, R.M., LEWERENZ, H.J., & ENGST, R. (1981) Electroneurophysiological studies on neurotoxic effects of hexachlorocyclohexane-isomers and gamma-pentachlorocyclohexane. Bull. environ. Contam. Toxicol., **27**: 704-706.

MURPHY, R. & HARVEY, C. (1985) Residues and metabolites of selected persistent halogenated hydrocarbons in blood specimens from a general population survey. Environ. Health Perspect., **60**: 115-120.

NAGASAKI, H. (1973) Chronic toxicity of benzene hexachloride (BHC). Nara Igaku Zasshi, **24**: 1-26.

NAGASAKI, H., KAWABATA, H., MIYATA, Y., INOUE, K., HIRAO, K., AOE, H., & ITO, N. (1975) Effect of various factors on induction of liver tumours in animals by the isomer of benzene hexachloride. Gann., 66: 185-191.

NAKAJIMA, E., SHINDO, H., & KURIHARA, N. (1970) [Whole body autoradiographic studies on the distribution of alpha-, beta-, and gamma-benzene hexachloride in mice.] Radio-isotopes, 19: 538 (in Japanese).

NIESSEN, K.H., RAMOLLAA, J., BINDER, M., BRUGMANN, G., & HOFMANN, U. (1984) Chlorinated hydrocarbons in adipose tissue of infants and toddlers: inventory and studies on their association with intake of mother's milk. Eur. J. Pediatr., 142: 238-243.

NIGAM, S.K., KARNIK, A.B., MAJUMDER, S.K., VISWESWARRIAH, K., SURYANARAYANA RAJU, G., MUKTHA BAI, K., LAKKAD, B.C., THAKORE, K.N., & CHATTERJEE, B.B. (1986) Serum hexachlorocyclohexane residues in workers engaged at a HCH manufacturing plant. Int. Arch. occup. environ. Health, 57: 315-320.

NISHIMURA, N. (1982) Survey on the mutagenicity of pesticides by a Salmonella microsome test. Aichi Ika Daigaku Igakkai Zasshi, 10(4): 305-312.

NOACK, G. & PORTIG, J. (1973) Biodegradation of alpha-hexachlorocyclohexane. III. Decrease in liver non-protein thiol after intragastric application of the drug. Naunyn-Schmiedebergs Arch. Pharmakol., 280: 183-189.

NOACK, G., PORTIG, J., & WIRSCHING, M. (1975) Biodegradation of alpha-hexachlorocyclohexane. IV. The extent of degradation of single doses in vivo. Naunyn-Schmiedebergs Arch. Pharmakol., 288: 57-64.

NOREN, K. (1983) Levels of organochlorine contaminants in human milk in relation to the dietary habits of the mothers. Acta paediatr. Scand., 72: 811-816.

NORSTROM, R.J., SIMON, M., MUIR, D.C.G., & SCHWEINSBURG, R.E. (1988) Organochlorine contaminants in Arctic marine food chains: Identification, geographical distribution and temporal trends in polar bears. Environ. Sci. Technol., 22: 1063-1071.

NYBOM, N. & KNUTSSON, B. (1947) Investigations on c-mitosis in *Allium cepa*. I. The cytological effect of hexachlorocyclohexane. Hereditas, 33: 220-234.

OEHME, M. & MANO (1984) The long-range transport of organic pollutants to the Arctic. Fresenius Z. anal. Chem., 319: 141-146.

OEHME, M. & STRAY, H. (1982) Quantitative determination of ultra-traces of chlorinated compounds in high-volume air samples from the Arctic using polyurethane foam as collecting medium. Fresenius Z. anal. Chem., 311: 665-673.

OSHIBA, K. (1972) Experimental studies on the fate of β- and γ-BHC *in vivo* following daily administration. Osaka Shiritsu Daigaku Igaku Zasshi, 21(1-3): 1-19.

References

OSHIBA, K. & KAWAKITA, H. (1972) Interaction between toxicant and nutrition. IV. Effect of lipid metabolism on reduction of the BHC deposition in rat tissues. Chem. Abstr., 77(8): 148231.

PALMER, C.M. & MALONEY, T.E. (1955) Preliminary screening for potential algicides. Ohio J. Sci., 55(1): 1-8.

POLISHUK, Z.W., WASSERMANN, M., WASSERMANN, D., GRONER, Y., LAZAROVICI, S., & TOMATIS, L. (1970) Effects of pregnancy on storage of organochlorine insecticides. Arch. environ. Health, 20: 215-217.

PORTIG, J. (1983) [Elimination of hexachlorocyclohexane (HCH) by mammals.] In: [Hexachlorocyclohexane as a harmful substance in foodstuffs. Papers from two seminars of the Senate Committee on the Testing of Residues in Foodstuffs held on 28-29 November 1979 and 6 March 1980], Weinheim, Chemie Verlag, pp. 108-118 (in German).

PORTIG, J. & VOHLAND, H.W. (1983) [Neuropharmacological and neurotoxic effects of hexachlorocyclohexane in man.] In: [Hexachlorocyclohexane as a harmful substance in foodstuffs. Papers from two seminars of the Senate Committee on the Testing of Residues in Foodstuffs held on 28-29 November 1979 and 6 March 1980], Weinheim, Chemie Verlag, pp. 215-226 (in German).

PORTIG, J., KRAUS, P., SODOMANN, S., & NOACK, G. (1973) Glutathion-dependent biotransformation in rats of isomers of hexachlorocyclohexane. Naunyn-Schmiedebergs Arch. Pharmakol., 279: 185-198.

PORTIG, J., STEIN, K., & VOHLAND, H.W. (1989) Preferential distribution of δ-hexachlorocyclohexane into cerebral white matter. Xenobiotica, 19(1): 123-130.

RADOMSKI, J.L., DEICHMANN, W.B., ALBERTO, A., REY, A., & MERKIN, T. (1971a) Human pesticide blood levels as a measure of body burden and pesticide exposure. Toxicol. appl. Pharmacol., 20: 175-185.

RADOMSKI, J.L., ASTOLFI, E., DEICHMANN, W.B., & REY, A.A. (1971b) Blood levels of organochlorine pesticides in Argentina. Occupationally and non-occupationally exposed adults, children, and new-born infants. Toxicol. appl. Pharmacol., 20: 186-193.

RAPPE, C., NYGREN, M., & LINDSTRÖM, G. (1987) Polychlorinated dibenzofurans and dibenzo-p-dioxins and other chlorinated contaminants in cow milk from various locations in Switzerland. Environ. Sci. Technol., 21: 964-970.

REINER, E., KRAUTHACKER, B., STIPCEVIC, M., & STEFANAC, Z. (1977) Blood levels of chlorinated hydrocarbon residues in the population of a continental town in Croatia (Yugoslavia). Pestic. monit. J., 11: 54-55.

RIEMSCHNEIDER, R. (1949) [A contribution to the toxicity of contact insecticides.] Anz. Schädlingskd., 22(1): 1-3 (in German).

SAGELSDORFF, P., LUTZ, W.K., & SCHLATTER, C. (1983) The relevance of covalent binding to mouse liver DNA to the carcinogenic action of hexachlorocyclohexane isomers. Carcinogenesis, 4(10): 1267-1273.

SAIKI, M.K. & SCHMITT, C.J. (1986) Organochlorine chemical residues in bluegills and common carp from the irrigated San Joaquin Valley Floor, California. Arch. environ. Contam. Toxicol., 15: 357-366.

SCHRÖTER, C., PARZEFALL, W., SCHRÖTER, H., & SCHULTE-HERMANN, R. (1987) Dose-response studies on the effects of α-, β-, and γ-hexachlorocyclohexane on putative preneoplastic foci, monooxygenases, and growth in rat liver. Cancer Res., 47: 80-88.

SCHULTE-HERMANN, R. & PARZEFALL, W. (1981) Failure to discriminate initiation from promotion of liver tumours in a long term study with the phenobarbital-type inducer alpha-hexachlorocyclohexane and the role of sustained stimulation of hepatic growth and monooxygenases. Cancer Res., 41: 4140-4146.

SCHULTE-HERMANN, R., LEBERL, C., LANDGRAF, H., & KORANSKY, W. (1974) Liver growth and mixed function oxidase activity: dose dependent stimulatory and inhibitory effects of alpha-hexachlorocyclohexane. Naunyn-Schmiedebergs Arch. exp. Pathol. Pharmakol., 285: 355-366.

SCHULTE-HERMANN, R., OHDE, G., SCHUPPLER, J., & TIMMERMANN-TROSIENER, I. (1981) Enhanced proliferation of putative preneoplastic cells in rat liver following treatment with the tumour promotors phenobarbital, hexachlorocyclohexane, steroid compounds and nafenopin. Cancer Res., 41(6): 2556-2562.

SCHULTE-HERMANN, R., TIMMERMANN-TROSIENER, I., & SCHUPPLER, J., (1983) Promotion of spontaneous preneoplastic cells in rat liver as a possible explanation of tumour production by non-mutagenic compounds. Cancer Res., 43: 839-844.

SEIFART, J. & BUCHAR, E. (1978) The biosynthesis of pyrimidine nucleotides and cytochrome P-450 content in rat liver microsomes after the administration of alpha-hexachlorocyclohexane (*in vivo* study). Toxicology, 11: 37-44.

SHAHIN, M. & VON BORSTEL, R. (1977) Mutagenic and lethal effects of alpha-benzene hexachloride, dibutyl phthalate and trichloroethylene in Saccharomyces cerevisiae. Mutat. Res., 48: 173-180.

SHAIN, W., NARANG, R., & SEEGAL, R. (1987) Neurotoxicity testing of chlorinated hydrocarbons by measuring specific neuronal and glial cell functions. Prog. clin. biol. Res., 253: 207-216.

SHIBATA, T. (1978) Experimental studies on the dynamic aspects of BHC and PCB *in vivo*. Jpn. J. Hyg., 32: 736-746.

SHIMAZU, H., SHIRAISHI, N., AKEMATSU, T., UEDA, N., & SUGIYAMA, T. (1976) Carcinogenicity screening tests on induction of chromosomal aberrations in rat bone marrow cells *in vivo*. Mutat. Res., 38: 347 (Abstract No. 20).

SIDDARAMAPPA, R. & SETHUNATHAN, N. (1975) Persistence of gamma-BHC and beta-BHC in Indian rice soils under flooded conditions. Pestic. Sci., 6: 395-403.

SIERRA, M. & SANTIAGO, D. (1987) Organochlorine pesticide levels in barn owls collected in Leon, Spain. Bull. environ. Contam. Toxicol., 38: 261-265.

References

SKAARE, J.U., TUVENG, J.M., & SANDE, H.A. (1988) Organochlorine pesticides and polychlorinated biphenyls in maternal adipose tissue, blood, milk, & cord blood from mothers and their infants living in Norway. Arch. environ. Toxicol., 17: 55-63.

SKAFTASON, J.F. & JOHANNESSON, T. (1979) Organochlorine compounds (DDT, hexachlorocyclohexane, hexachlorobenzene) in Icelandic animal body fat and butter fat: Local and global sources of contamination. Acta pharmacol. toxicol., 44: 156-157.

SLOOFF, W. & MATTHIJSEN, A.J.C.M. (1988) Integrated criteria document: Hexachlorocyclohexanes, Bilthoven, National Institute of Public Health and Environmental Protection (Report No. 758473011).

SRINIVASAN, K. & RADHAKRISHNAMURTY, R. (1977) Effect of beta- and gamma-isomers of hexachlorocyclohexane on some liver and kidney enzymes in albino rats. Curr. Sci., 46: 598-600.

SRINIVASAN, K. & RADHAKRISHNAMURTY, R. (1983) Studies on the distribution of the beta- and gamma-isomers of hexachlorocyclohexane in rat tissues. J. environ. Sci. Health, B18(3): 401-418.

SRINIVASAN, K. & RADHAKRISHNAMURTY, R. (1988) Biochemical changes produced by beta- and gamma-Hexachlorocyclohexane isomers in albino rats. J. environ. Sci. Health, B23(4): 367-386.

SRINIVASAN, K., RAMESH, H.P., & RADHAKRISHNAMURTY, R. (1984) Renal tubular dysfunction caused by dietary hexachlorocyclohexane (HCH) isomers. J. environ. Sci. Health, B19(45): 453-466.

SRINIVASAN, K., RAMESH, H.P., & RADHAKRISHNAMURTY, R. (1988) Changes induced by hexachlorocyclohexane isomers in rat livers and testes. Bull. environ. Contam. Toxicol., 41: 531-539.

STARR, H.G., Jr, ALDRICH, F.D., MCDOUGALL, W.D., III, & MOUNCE, L.M. (1974) Contribution of household dust to the human exposure to pesticides. Pestic. monit. J., 8: 209-212.

STEIN, K. & PORTIG, J. (1976) Oxidative transformation of hexachlorocyclohexane in the rat. Naunyn-Schmiedebergs Arch. Pharmacol., 293: R51.

STEIN, K., PORTIG, J., & KORANSKY, W. (1977) Oxidative transformation of hexachlorocyclohexane in rats and with rat liver microsomes. Naunyn-Schmiedebergs Arch. Pharmakol., 298: 115-128.

STEIN, K., PORTIG, J., FUHRMANN, H., KORANSKY, W., & NOACK, G. (1980) Steric factors in the pharmacokinetics of lindane and α-hexachlorocyclohexane in rats. Xenobiotica, 10(1): 65-77.

STRACHAN, W.M.J., HUNEAULT, H., SCHERTZER, W.M., & ELDER, F.C. (1980) Organochlorines in precipitation in the Great Lakes Region. In: Afghan, B.K. & MacKay, D., ed. Hydrocarbons and halogenated hydrocarbons in the aquatic environment, New York, London, Plenum Press.

SUGIURA, K., SATO, S., GOTO, M., & KURIHARA, Y. (1976) Effects of beta-HCH on aquatic microcosm. Chemosphere, 1: 39-44.

SUGIURA, K., WASHINO, T., HATTORI, M., SATO, E., & GOTO, M. (1979) Accumulation of organochlorine compounds in fishes. Difference of accumulation factors by fishes. Chemosphere, 6: 359-364.

SUZUKI, M., YAMATO, Y., & WATANABE, T. (1975) Persistence of BHC (1,2,3,4,5,6-hexachlorocyclohexane) and dieldrin residues in field soils. Bull. environ. Contam. Toxicol., 14(5): 520-529.

SZOKOLAY, A., ROSIVAL, L., UHNAK, J., & MADARIC, A. (1977a) Dynamics of benzene hexachloride (BHC) isomers and other chlorinated pesticides in the food chain and human fat. Ecotoxicol. environ. Saf., 1(1): 349-359.

SZOKOLAY, A., MADARIC, A., & UHNAK, J. (1977b) Relative cumulation of beta-HCH in ecological and biological systems. J. environ. Sci. Health, B12(3): 193-212.

SZYMCZYNSKI, G.A., WALISZEWSKI, S.M., TUSZEWSKI, M., & PYDA, P. (1986) Chlorinated pesticides levels in human adipose tissue in the district of Poznan. J. environ. Sci. Health, A21(1): 5-14.

TAKABATAKE, E. (1978) Levels of organochlorine compounds and heavy metals in tissues of the general population in Japan. Geogr. med., 8: 1-23.

TANABE, S., TATSUKAWA, R., KAWANO, M., & HIDAKA, H. (1982) Global distribution and atmospheric transport of chlorinated hydrocarbons: HCH(BHC) isomers and DDT compounds in the Western Pacific, Eastern Indian- and Antarctic Oceans. J. Oceanogr. Soc. Jpn, 38(3): 137-148.

TANOOKA, H. (1977) Development and applications of *Bacillus subtilis* test systems for mutagens, involving DNA-repair deficiency and suppressible auxotrophic mutations. Mutat. Res., 42: 19-32.

THAMAVIT, W., HIASA, Y., ITO, N., & BHAMARA-PRAVATI, N. (1974) The inhibitory effects of alpha-benzene hexachloride on 3'-methyl-4-dimethyl amino-benzene and DL-ethionine carcinogenesis in rats. Cancer Res., 34: 337-340.

THORPE, E. & WALKER, A.I.T. (1973) The toxicology of dieldrin (HEOD). II Comparative long-term oral toxicity studies in mice with dieldrin, DDT, phenobarbitone, β-BHC and γ-BHC. Food Cosmet. Toxicol., 11: 433-442.

TIECCO, G. (1961) [Testing for synthetic oestrogens in foodstuffs.] Vet. Ital., 12: 447-460 (in Italian).

TOMCZAK, S., BAUMANN, K., & LEHNERT, G. (1981) Occupational exposure to hexachlorocyclohexane. IV. Sex hormone alterations in HCH-exposed workers. Int. Arch. occup. environ. Health, 48: 283-287.

TRYPHONAS, L. & IVERSON, F. (1983) Sequential histopathologic analysis of α-hexachlorocyclohexane induced hepatic megalocytosis and adenoma formation in the HPB mouse. J. Natl Cancer Inst., 71(6): 1307-1318.

TSUKANO, Y. (1973) Factors affecting disappearance of BHC-isomers from rice field soil. Jpn. agric. Res. Q., 7(2): 93-97.

TUINSTRA, L.G.M.Th. (1971) Organochlorine insecticide residues in human milk in the Leiden region. Neth. Milk Dairy J., 25: 24-32.

UMWELTBUNDESAMT (1989) [Data on the environment, 1988/89], Berlin, Schmidt E. Verlag, pp. 403-405, 410-412, 416-417, 521-522, 524, 526 (in German).

VAN ASPEREN, K. (1954) Interaction of the isomers of benzenehexachloride in mice. Arch. Int. Pharmacodyn., 99(3/4): 368-377.

VAN GIERSBERGEN, P.L.M., VAN VELSEN, F.L., VAN LEEUWEN, F.X.R., & DANSE, L.H.J.C. (1984) [Toxicity of beta-HCH: relationship between the biochemistry and pathology of the liver in a 6-week feeding test], Bilthoven, National Institute of Public Health and Environmental Hygiene (Unpublished report No. 618303001) (in Dutch).

VAN HOOF, M., VAN VELSEN, F.L., DANSE, L.H.J.C., & VAN LEEUWEN, F.X.R. (1982) [Toxicity of beta-HCH: relationship between the biochemistry and pathology of the liver in a 3-week feeding test], Bilthoven, National Institute of Public Health and Environmental Hygiene (Report No. 618115001) (in Dutch).

VAN VELSEN, F.L. (1986) The oestrogenicity of the environmental contaminant β-hexachlorocyclohexane, University of Utrecht (Thesis).

VAN VELSEN, F.L., VAN LEEUWEN, F.X.R., & DANSE, L.H.J.C. (1982) [Investigation into the toxicity, kinetics and metabolism of beta- and gamma-HCH], Bilthoven, National Institute of Public Health and Environmental Hygiene (Unpublished report No. 617908003) (in Dutch).

VAN VELSEN, F.L., DANSE, L.H.J.C., VAN LEEUWEN, F.X.R., DORMANS, J.A.M.A., & VAN LOGTEN, M.J. (1986) The subchronic oral toxicity of the β-isomer of hexachlorocyclohexane in rats. Fundam. appl. Toxicol., 6: 697-712.

VOHLAND, H.W., PORTIG, J., & STEIN, K. (1981) Neuropharmacological effects of isomers of hexachlorocyclohexane. 1. Protection against pentylenetetrazol-induced convulsions. Toxicol. appl. Pharmacol., 57(3): 425-438.

VOHLAND, H.W. & KORANSKY, W. (1983) [The behaviour and effects of hexachlorocyclohexane in man.] In: [Hexachlorocyclohexane as a harmful substance in foodstuffs. Paper from two seminars of the Senate Committee on the Testing of Residues in Foodstuffs held on 28-29 November 1979 and 6 March 1980], Weinheim, Chemie Verlag, pp. 246-262 (in German).

VUKAVIC, T., PAVKOV, S., CUSIC, S., RONCEVIC, N., VOJINOVIC, M., & TOKOVIC, B. (1986) Pesticide residues in human colostrum: seasonal variations, Yugoslavia. Arch. environ. Contam. Toxicol., 15: 525-528.

WAHID, P.A. & SETHUNATHAN, N. (1979) Sorption-desorption of α, β, and γ isomers of hexachlorocyclohexane in soils. J. agric. food Chem., 27(5): 1050-1053.

WASSERMANN, M., ROGOFF, M.G., TOMATIS, L., DAY, N.E., WASSERMANN, D., DJAVAHERIAN, M., & GUTTEL, C. (1972) Storage of organochlorine insecticides in the adipose tissue of people in Kenya. Ann. Soc. Belge Méd. Trop., 52(6): 509-514.

WEGMAN, R.C.C. & GREVE, P.A. (1980) Halogenated hydrocarbons in Dutch water samples over the years 1969-1977. In: Afghan, B.K. & MacKay, D., ed. Hydrocarbons and halogenated hydrocarbons in the aquatic environment, New York, London, Plenum Press, pp. 405-415.

WESTER, P.W. & CANTON, J.H. (1986) Histopathological study of *Oryzias latipes* (medaka) after long-term β-hexachlorocyclohexane exposure. Aquat. Toxicol., 9: 21-45.

WESTER, P.W., CANTON, J.H., & BISSCHOP, A. (1985) Histopathological study of *Poecilia reticulata* (guppy) after long-term β-hexachlorocyclohexane exposure. Aquat. Toxicol., 6: 271-296.

WHO (1986) Joint FAO/WHO Food Contamination Monitoring Programme. Summary of 1980-1983 monitoring data, Geneva, World Health Organization (GEMS report WHO/EHE/FOS/86.2).

WHO (1991) Environmental Health Criteria 124: Lindane, Geneva, World Health Organization.

WITTICH, U. & SCHULTE-HERMANN, R. (1977) Liver growth and hepatic monooxygenase activity in suckling rats following administration of alpha-hexachlorocyclohexane to the mother. Arch. Pharmacol., 297(suppl. II): R15.

WITTLINGER, R. & BALLSCHMITER, K. (1987) Global baseline pollution studies XI: Congener specific determination of polychlorinated biphenyls (PCBs) and occurrence of alpha- and gamma-hexachlorocyclohexane (HCH), 4.4'-DDE and 4.4'-DDT in continental air. Chemosphere, 16(10/12): 2497-2513.

WOLF, H.P. (1983) [Implementation of results of a trial with dairy cows contaminated with 12-HCH.] In: [Hexachlorocyclohexane as a harmful substance in foodstuffs. Papers from two seminars of the Senate Committee on the Testing of Residues in Foodstuffs held on 28-29 November 1979 and 6 March 1980], Weinheim, Chemie Verlag, pp. 143-154 (in German).

YAMATO, Y., KIYONAGA, M., & WATANABE, T. (1983) Comparative bioaccumulation and elimination of HCH-isomers in short-necked clam *(Venerupis japonica)* and guppy *(Poecilia reticulata)*. Bull. environ. Contam. Toxicol., 31: 352-359.

ZHOU, X., LIU, R., ZHANG, W., XUE, X., & LIU, H. (1986) The effect of BHC isomers on photosynthetic formation of oxygen by green algae. Zhiwu Shenglixue Tongxun, 6: 32-34.

APPENDIX 1. CHEMICAL STRUCTURE

The basic structure of HCH is a closed chain of six carbon atoms. The structure can have two spatial forms, i.e. cis and trans configurations. Every carbon atom is bound to a hydrogen and a chlorine atom. One of these substituents forms a plane with the two connecting carbon atoms. Since this plane parallels the "equator" of the molecule, this atom is said to be in the equatorial position. The binding with the other atom parallels the "axis" of the molecule. Therefore, this one is in the axial position. Due to the size of the chlorine atom the carbon atoms are not free to rotate. Hence the positions of the chlorine and hydrogen atoms are fixed, one being always in the equatorial position and the other in the axial position.

The various combinations of the spatial orientation of the hydrogen and chlorine atoms on each of the carbon atoms of cyclohexane results in different isomeric compounds. Theoretically, 17 isomers of HCH are possible, but, due to spatial incompatibilities and thermodynamic instability, only nine isomers have in fact been detected. They all have the trans configuration.

In the beta-isomer, all chlorine atoms are in the equatorial position.

The positions of the chlorine atoms in the major isomers of HCH are presented in Table 9 (Demozay & Marechal, 1972; Van Velsen, 1986).

Table 9. Positions of chlorine atoms in the major HCH isomers

Isomer	Chlorine positions[b]	Physical structure
Alpha[a]	A A E E E E	monoclinic prisms
Beta	E E E E E E	octahedral cubic crystals
Gamma	A A A E E E	monoclinic crystals
Delta	A E E E E E	crystals/fine platelets
Epsilon	A E E A E E	monoclinic needles or hexagonal monoclinic crystals

[a] racemate of two optical isomers
[b] A = axial position; E = equatorial position   From: van Velsen (1986).

RESUME ET EVALUATION

1. Alpha-hexachlorocyclohexane

1.1 Propriétés générales

L'Alpha-hexachlorocyclohexane (alpha-HCH) est un important sous-produit (60-70%) de la fabrication du lindane (> 99% de gamma-HCH). Il est peu soluble dans l'eau mais très soluble dans les solvants organiques comme l'acétone, le chloroforme et le xylène. C'est un solide de faible tension de vapeur. Son coefficient de partage entre le n-octanol et l'eau (log P_{ow}) est de 3,82. C'est un polluant de l'environnement.

L'alpha-HCH peut être dosé séparément des autres isomères par chromatographie en phase gazeuse avec détection par capture d'électrons ou par d'autres méthodes après extraction par partage liquide/liquide et purification sur colonne chromatographique.

1.2 Transport, distribution et transformation dans l'environnement

Il se produit dans l'environnement une biodégradation ainsi qu'une dégradation abiotique (déchloration) sous l'action du rayonnement ultraviolet, qui aboutissent respectivement, au delta-3,4,5,6-tétrachlohéxène et au pentachlorocyclohéxène Ce processus de décomposition est plus lent que dans le cas du lindane. La persistance de l'alpha-HCH dans le sol dépend de facteurs environnementaux comme l'action des microorganismes, la teneur en matières organiques, la co-distillation et l'évaporation. Il n'y a pas d'isomérisation du lindane en alpha-HCH.

La bioconcentration est rapide chez les microorganismes (facteur de bioconcentration allant de 1500 à 2700, calculé en poids à sec ou environ 12 000 calculé par rapport aux lipides en l'espace de 30 minutes): chez les invertébrés, il est de 60 à 2750 (poids à sec) ou > 8000 (par rapport aux lipides) sur une durée de 24 à 72 heures. Dans le cas des poissons ces chiffres vont de 313 à 1216 sur 4 à 28 jours, les valeurs pouvant atteindre 50 000 pour les poissons de l'Elbe. Toutefois la biotransformation et l'élimination sont également assez rapide chez ces organismes (15 minutes à 72 heures).

1.3 Concentrations dans l'environnement et exposition humaine

L'alpha-HCH est présent dans l'air des océans à la concentration de 0,02 à 1,5 mg/m^3. Au Canada, on en a trouvé dans l'eau de pluie à des teneurs de 1 à 40 ng par litre, mais la neige n'en contenait que des traces.

Au cours de la période 1969-1974, on a constaté dans le Rhin et ses affluents des concentrations d'alpha-HCH comprises entre 0,01 et 2,7 µg/litre; toutefois, plus récemment, ces concentrations sont descendues en-dessous de 0,01 µg/litre. Dans l'Elbe, les concentrations sont passées de 0,023 µg/litre en moyenne en 1981, à moins de 0,012 µg/litre en 1988. Dans un certain nombre de cours d'eau du Royaume-Uni on a trouvé en 1966 des concentrations allant de 0,001 à 0,43 µg/litre. En Frise, dans le nord de la Mer des Wadden on a trouvé dans les sédiments des concentrations d'alpha-HCH allant de 0,3 à 1,4 µg/kg (0,002 µg/litre d'eau).

Les teneurs en alpha-HCH de différentes espèces végétales en provenance de divers pays vont de 0,5 à 2140 µg/kg de poids sec mais elles peuvent être encore beaucoup plus élevées dans les régions polluées. Même dans l'Antarctique, on a rencontré des concentrations allant de 0,2 à 1,15 µg/kg.

On trouve régulièrement du alpha-HCH dans les poissons et les invertébrés aquatiques ainsi que chez des canards, des hérons et des effraies. On a trouvé dans la graisse sous-cutanée de rennes et d'orignaux vivant dans des régions où l'épandage de pesticides est négligeable, des quantités d'alpha-HCH égales en moyenne à 7-80 µg/kg. Dans les tissus adipeux d'ours polaires canadiens on a trouvé des teneurs d'alpha-HCH allant de 0,3 à 0,87 mg/kg (calculées par rapport au tissu adipeux).

Dans un certain nombre de pays on a procédé à l'analyse de denrées alimentaires importantes à la recherche d'alpha-HCH. Les teneurs mesurées, présentes essentiellement dans des produits contenant des graisses, allaient jusqu'à 0,05 mg/kg de produit, sauf dans le lait et les produits laitiers (jusqu'à 0,22 mg/kg) et dans le poisson et les produits carnés industriels (jusqu'à 0,5 mg/kg par rapport aux graisses). On a constaté un léger recul des teneurs au cours des années.

C'est principalement par les aliments que la population dans son ensemble est exposée à l'alpha-HCH. Des études de ration totale effectuées aux Pays-Bas et au Royaume-Uni ont révélé des concentrations moyennes respectivement égales à 0,01 et 0,002-0,003 mg/kg. Les données concernant le Royaume-Uni montrent qu'il existe une tendance à la baisse depuis 1967. Aux Etats-Unis d'Amérique, l'apport alimentaire moyen d'alpha-HCH a été de 0,09 à 0,025 mg/kg de poids corporel par jour, au cours de la période 1977-1979 et de 0,003 à 0,016 µg/kg de poids corporel au cours de la période 1982-1984.

Dans quelques pays, on a mesuré la concentration d'alpha-HCH dans le sang, le sérum et le plasma humain. La concentration moyenne (dans certains cas, la médiane) était inférieure à 0,1 µg/litre (intervalle de variation: de non décelable à 0,6 µg/litre). Dans un des pays cependant on a relevé une concentration moyenne de 3,5 µg/litre (intervalle de variation 0,1 à 15,0) dans le tiers environ des échantillons de sang.

Dans le tissu adipeux humain et le lait maternel, les concentrations d'alpha-HCH qui ont été relevées sont faibles (respectivement moins de 0,01-0,1 et moins de 0,001-0,04 mg/kg calculées par rapport aux graisses). Des études de ration totale ont montré que l'apport alimentaire quotidien était de l'ordre de 0,01 µg/kg de poids corporel ou moins. Ces concentrations ont tendance à diminuer avec le temps.

L'alpha-HCH se présente comme un contaminant universel de l'environnement. Les teneurs ne diminuent que lentement malgré les mesures prises en vue d'en éviter la propagation dans le milieu.

1.4 Cinétique et métabolisme

Chez le rat, l'alpha-HCH est rapidement et presque complètement résorbé au niveau des voies digestives. Après injection intrapéritonéale, environ 40 à 80% de l'alpha-HCH administré a été excrété dans les urines et 50 à 20% dans les matières fécales. Chez le rat également, les concentrations les plus élevées se rencontrent dans le foie, les reins, les tissus adipeux, l'encéphale et les muscles, avec une accumulation importante dans la fraction lipidique. On a constaté que chez des rats à la mamelle, la concentration hépatique d'alpha-HCH était deux fois plus élevée que chez les mères. Chez le rat également, le rapport de la concentration dans l'encéphale à la concentration sanguine et de la concentration dans la masse grasse à la concentration sanguine était respectivement de 120:1 et 397:1.

Chez le rat, la biotransformation de l'alpha-HCH comporte une déchloration. Le principal métabolite urinaire est le 2,4,6-trichlorophénol; on a également identifié d'autres métabolites tels que le 1,2,4, le 2,3,4 et le 2,4,5-trichlorophénol ainsi que le 2,3,4,5- et le 2,3,4,6-tétrachlorophénol. On a trouvé dans les reins de rats du 1,3,4,5,6-pentachlorocyhex-1-ène, substance dont la présence a été également observée dans le foie de poulets lors d'études *in vitro.* Dans le foie, il y a conjugaison avec le glutathion.

Le demi-vie de libération à partir de la masse grasse est de 6,9 jours chez la ratte et de 1,6 jour chez le rat.

1.5 Effets sur les êtres vivants dans leur milieu naturel

L'alpha-HCH est faiblement toxique pour les algues, la dose sans effet observable se situant en général à 2 mg/litre.

Une étude de longue durée sur *Daphnia magna* a montré que la dose sans effet observable était de 0,05 mg/litre pour cette espèce. L'alpha-HCH est modérément toxique pour les invertébrés et les poissons. Pour ces organismes, les valeurs de la $CL(E)_{50}$ sont de l'ordre de 1 mg/litre. Lors d'études de courte durée effectuées sur des guppies et sur *Oryzia latipes,* on a constaté qu'une dose de 0,8 mg/litre était sans effet.

Lors d'études de trois mois sur *Salmo gairdneri* soumis à des doses allant de 10 à 1250 mg/kg de nourriture, on n'a observé aucun effet sur la mortalité, le comportement, la croissance ou l'activité enzymatique du foie et du cerveau.

Des études de courte et de longue durée sur un mollusque *(Lymnea stagnalis)* ont montré que la CE_{50} était dans ce cas de 1200 µg/litre (déterminée d'après la mortalité et l'immobilisation des mollusques). A la concentration de 250 µg/litre il y a eu inhibition de la ponte. Une réduction de 50% a été notée dans le taux global de reproduction à la concentration de 65 µg/litre.

On ne dispose d'aucune donnée concernant les effets sur les populations et les écosystèmes.

1.6 Effets sur les animaux d'expérience et les systèmes d'épreuve in vitro

La DL_{50} se situe entre 1000 et 4000 mg/kg pour la souris et entre 500 et 4670 mg/kg de poids corporel pour le rat. Les signes d'intoxication sont essentiellement ceux d'une stimulation du système nerveux central.

Lors d'une étude de 90 jours sur des rats, on a constaté une baisse de la croissance à la concentration de 250 mg/kg de nourriture. A partir de 50 mg/kg, des modifications au niveau histologique et enzymatique témoignaient d'une induction des enzymes. A ces doses on a également noté des signes d'immunodépression. Il y avait déjà accroissement du poids du foie à partir de 10 mg/kg de nourriture (soit l'équivalent de 0,5 mg/kg de poids corporel). La dose sans effet nocif observé se situait à 2 mg/kg de nourriture (soit l'équivalent de 0,1 mg/kg de poids corporel par jour).

Il n'y a pas eu d'études convenables de toxicité à long terme ni d'études sur la reproduction et le pouvoir tératogène.

Des études effectuées sur diverses souches de *Salmonella typhimurium* n'ont révélé aucun signe de mutagénicité, que ce soit en présence ou en l'absence d'une activation métabolique. Les tests sur *Saccharomyces cerevisiae* ont également été négatifs, toutefois la recherche d'une synthèse non programmée de l'ADN sur des hépatocytes de rat *in vitro* a donné un résultat équivoque.

On a effectué des travaux en vue de déterminer le pouvoir cancérogène de l'alpha-HCH sur des rats et des souris à des doses allant de 100 à 600 mg/kg de nourriture. Chez des souris, on a observé des nodules hyperplastiques et/ou des adénomes hépatocellulaires. Dans une des études, les doses dépassaient la dose maximale tolérable. Lors de trois autres études, deux sur des souris et une sur des rats, on n'a observé aucune augmentation dans l'incidence des tumeurs à des doses allant jusqu'à 160 mg/kg de nourriture (souris) et 640 mg/kg de nourriture (rats).

Les résultats des études sur le pouvoir d'initiation et de promotion ainsi que sur le mode d'action de l'alpha-HCH, de même que les tests de mutagénicité, montrent que les tumeurs induites par l'alpha-HCH chez la souris ne sont pas d'origine génétique.

On a montré que l'alpha-HCH provoquait une nette augmentation de l'activité des enzymes hépatiques, même à des doses de 5 mg/kg de nourriture (soit l'équivalent de 0,25 mg/kg de poids corporel). A la dose de 2 mg/kg de poids corporel, l'alpha-HCH n'a eu aucun effet sur la déméthylation de l'aminopyrine ni sur la teneur du foie en ADN.

1.7 Effets sur l'homme

L'examen de travailleurs d'une usine produisant du lindane, qui avaient été exposés pendant 7,2 années (en moyenne géométrique, avec des limites de 1 à 30 ans), a permis de conclure qu'une exposition professionnelle au HCH ne produit pas de signes de troubles neurologiques ni de perturbation de la fonction neuromusculaire.

RESUME ET EVALUATION

2. Béta-hexachlorocyclohexane

2.1 Propriétés générales

Le béta-hexachlorocyclohexane (béta-HCH) est un sous-produit (7-10%) de la fabrication du lindane (> de 99% de gamma-HCH). Peu soluble dans l'eau, il est très soluble dans les solvants organiques tels que l'acétone, le cyclohexane et xylène. C'est un solide de faible tension de vapeur. Son coefficient de partage entre le n-octanol et l'eau (log P_{ow}) est égal à 3,80. C'est un polluant de l'environnement.

On peut doser le béta-HCH séparément des autres isomères par chromatographie en phase gazeuse avec détection par capture d'électrons ainsi que par d'autres méthodes après extraction par partage liquide/liquide et purification sur colonne chromatographique.

2.2 Transport, distribution et transformation dans l'environnement

La biodégradation et la dégradation abiotique (déchloration) sous l'effet du rayonnement ultraviolet, produisent du pentachlorocyclohexane, mais beaucoup plus lentement que dans le cas du lindane (gamma-HCH).

Le béta-HCH est l'isomère le plus persistant de l'HCH. Sa persistance dans le sol dépend de facteurs environnementaux tels que l'action des microorganismes, la teneur en matières organiques et en eau ainsi que la co-distillation et l'évaporation.

En raison de sa persistance, le béta-HCH subit une bioconcentration rapide chez les invertébrés (le facteur de bioconcentration est d'environ 125 en l'espace de trois jours), chez les poissons (250-1500 calculé à partir du poids à sec ou environ 500 000 fois calculé sur la base des lipides en l'espace de 3 à 10 minutes), ainsi que chez les oiseaux et l'homme (environ 525). Le béta-HCH se concentre davantage et s'élimine plus lentement que les autres isomères de l'HCH.

2.3 Concentrations dans l'environnement et exposition humaine

On rencontre le béta-HCH dans l'air des océans à des concentrations de 0,004 à 0,13 ng/m^3.

Jusqu'en 1974, le Rhin et ses affluents présentaient des teneurs en béta-HCH allant de 0,14 à 0,22 µg par litre, mais depuis on constate que ces valeurs sont systématiquement inférieures à 0,12 µg/litre. Des échantillons prélevés dans la Meuse présentaient des teneurs inférieures à 0,12 µg/litre. Dans l'Elbe, les concentrations sont passées en moyenne de 0,009 à 0,004 µg/litre entre 1981 et 1988.

On a dosé le béta-HCH chez des oiseaux tels que les éperviers, les faucons crécerelles, les hiboux, les hérons et les grèbes pendant un certain nombre d'années et l'on a observé des concentrations allant de 0,1 à 0,3 mg/kg. Chez les ours polaires on a mesuré des concentrations allant jusqu'à 0,87 mg/kg (par rapport au tissu adipeux) dans le foie et les graisses.

Dans quelques pays on a procédé à l'analyse de denrées alimentaires importantes en vue d'y rechercher la présence de béta-HCH. Les concentrations moyennes, mesurées essentiellement dans des denrées contenant des graisses, allaient jusqu'à 0.03 mg/kg (par rapport au contenu lipidique), mais on en a trouvé jusqu'à 4 mg/kg (par rapport au contenu lipidique) dans des produits laitiers. Dans les denrées non grasses, les teneurs étaient inférieures à 0,05 mg/kg de produit. En général, ces teneurs sont en lent recul.

C'est principalement par les aliments que la population dans son ensemble est exposée au béta-HCH. Lors d'études de ration totale effectuées au Royaume-Uni, on a mesuré des concentrations de 0,003, 0,0005 et moins de 0,0005 mg/kg respectivement en 1966/67, 1975/77 et 1981. Aux Etats-Unis d'Amérique, l'apport moyen quotidien d'origine alimentaire allait en 1982-84 de moins de 0,1 à 0,4 ng/kg de poids corporel dans les différents groupes d'âge.

Dans un certain nombre de pays, on a procédé au dosage du béta-HCH dans le sang, le sérum ou le plasma au sein de la population générale. Les concentrations varient d'un pays à l'autre, atteignant parfois 25 µg/litre.

De nombreuses études ont été menées afin de rechercher la présence de béta-HCH dans les tissus adipeux humains. Les concentrations relevées au Canada, en République fédérale d'Allemagne, au Kenya, aux Pays-Bas et au Royaume-Uni atteignaient jusqu'à 4,4 mg/kg (par rapport au contenu lipidique). On a constaté une augmentation progressive avec l'âge jusqu'à environ 50 ans, après quoi les teneurs déclinaient. Dans les tissus adipeux, les concentrations de béta-HCH sont plus élevées que celles des autres isomères, phénomène qui traduit la tendance à l'accumulation de cette substance. Il n'y a pas de tendance claire à la baisse des concentrations de béta-HCH sur la période au cours de laquelle ces études ont été effectuées. On a constaté l'existence d'une relation entre les concentrations de béta-HCH dans les tissus adipeux et le lait maternel d'une part, et la consommation de produits carnés, de graisses animales et de poissons gras, d'autre part.

Dans quelques pays (Canada, République fédérale d'Allemagne, Pays-Bas et Royaume-Uni) on a procédé au dosage du béta-HCH dans le lait maternel et obtenu des concentrations allant de 0,1 à 0,69 mg/kg (par rapport au contenu lipidique). Il ressort de ces analyses que la concentration du béta-HCH est plus élevée dans le lait des femmes des zones rurales que dans celui des femmes des zones urbaines.

Le béta-HCH apparaît comme un contaminant universel de l'environnement. Les concentrations n'accusent qu'une très lente tendance à la baisse malgré les mesures prises en vue d'en empêcher la propagation dans l'environnement.

2.4 Cinétique et métabolisme

Le béta-HCH est absorbé jusqu'à 95% dans les voies digestives de la souris, et s'accumule ensuite en majeure partie dans les tissus adipeux. L'élimination s'effectue selon un mécanisme en deux étapes, la demi-vie étant de 2,5 jours pour la première et de 18 jours pour la seconde.

Une fois résorbé, le béta-HCH se répartit rapidement dans les divers organes et tissus: foie, encéphale, reins et tissus adipeux. Chez le rat, la concentration maximale dans le foie est atteinte en quatre jours. Pour une concentration sanguine moyenne de 92 µg/litre (mais également pour des concentrations de 540 et 2100 µg/litre), le rapport des concentrations dans le cerveau et le sang d'une part et dans le tissu adipeux et le sang d'autre part était respectivement de 2:1 et de 170:1. Après une intoxication mortelle chez l'homme par des isomères de l'HCH, on a constaté que la concentration en béta-HCH mesurée par rapport à la teneur du sang était de 363 dans les tissus adipeux, de 3 dans le cerveau et de 15 dans le foie. Le béta-HCH franchit la barrière hémo-méningée beaucoup moins facilement que les autres isomères de l'HCH.

Chez des souris gravides, le passage transplacentaire du béta-HCH au foetus était d'environ 2% de la dose, mais atteignait 40% chez des rattes gravides. Chez le rat, le passage de la mère aux ratons à la mamelle par l'intermédiaire du lait correspondait à environ 60% de la dose.

Chez le rat, 70% du béta-HCH est éliminé dans les 28 premiers jours, dont un tiers par la voie urinaire. On ne retrouve pas de béta-HCH inchangé dans l'urine. Le principal métabolite résultant de la cis-déshydrochloration est le 2,4,6-trichlorophénol sous forme conjuguée.

Un prétraitement au moyen de béta-HCH modifie le métabolisme du lindane chez le rat. D'après des études comportant l'administration de béta-HCH par voie intrapéritonéale à des souris, il semble que celui-ci soit métabolisé plus lentement que le lindane.

2.5 Effets sur les êtres vivants dans leur milieu naturel

En général le béta-HCH est modérément toxique pour les algues, les invertébrés et les poissons. La DL_{50} aiguë pour ces organismes est de l'ordre de 1 mg/litre mais les valeurs de la CE_{50} sont plus faibles (0,05-0,5 mg/litre). Dans le cas de deux espèces de poisson d'eau douce, *Oryzia latipes* et *Poecilia reticulata*, la dose sans effet observable a été fixée à 0,03 mg/litre sur une durée de un et trois mois respectivement.

On ne dispose d'aucune donnée concernant les effets sur les populations et les écosystèmes.

2.6 Effets sur les animaux d'expérience et les systèmes d'épreuve in vitro

Les valeurs de la DL_{50} aiguë par voie orale pour les souris et les rats publiées en 1968, se situaient entre 1500 et 2000 mg/kg de poids corporel. Toutefois des études plus récentes ont fourni des valeurs de 16 g/kg de poids corporel pour les souris et de 8 g/kg de poids corporel pour les rats. Les signes d'intoxication sont essentiellement neurologiques.

Des études de courte durée sur des souris avec des doses allant jusqu'à 600 mg/kg de nourriture pendant 26 à 32 semaines, ont révélé la présence d'une hyperplasie nodulaire et de proliférations atypiques au niveau du foie ainsi qu'une augmentation du poids de cet organe. Lors d'une troisième étude, consistant dans l'administration de doses allant jusqu'à 500 mg/kg de nourriture pendant 24 semaines, on a observé ni tumeurs hépatiques ni hyperplasie nodulaire.

Une étude de 90 jours au cours de laquelle des rats ont reçu soit 50 soit 250 mg de béta-HCH par kg de nourriture, a révélé des altérations au niveau du foie, notamment une hypertrophie et une prolifération du réticulum endoplasmique lisse ainsi qu'un accroissement de l'activité des enzymes microsomiques. Aux doses les plus élevées on a également observé des altérations au niveau des gonades qui s'accompagnaient également d'effets graves sur le poids du corps. Les modifications hormonales accompagnant l'atrophie des gonades ne correspondaient pas à un effet endocrinien systématique. Aucun effet nocif n'a été constaté à la dose de 2 mg/kg de nourriture (soit l'équivalent de 0,1 mg/kg de poids corporel).

Une étude de longue durée sur des rats (publiée en 1950) au cours de laquelle on a administré des doses de 10 mg/kg de nourriture (soit l'équivalent de 0,5 mg/kg de poids corporel) ou davantage, a révélé que ce régime conduisait à une hypertrophie du foie et à des modifications histologiques.

Lors d'une étude de reproduction portant sur deux générations de rats, on a observé les mêmes effets que dans l'étude de 90 jours citée plus haut. Aucun effet n'a été observé à la dose de 2 mg/kg de nourriture (soit l'équivalent de 0,1 mg/kg de poids corporel), mais à la dose de 10 mg/kg, il y avait accroissement de la mortalité et de la stérilité. L'étude a également porté sur les effets tératogènes éventuels du béta-HCH mais aucun effet de ce genre imputable au produit n'a été observé.

On a décrit un effet "oestrogénique" faible dont l'organe cible serait l'utérus. En fait il n'y a pas d'effet bien net sur le système de régulation endocrinienne. Le mécanisme et la portée de cet effet demeurent incertains.

Les études de mutagénicité publiées ne font état d'aucune augmentation dans la fréquence des mutations chez les souches de *Salmonella typhimurium*. Une étude *in vivo* chez le rat sur des cellules de moelle osseuse en métaphase a donné des résultats positifs.

Deux études ont été effectuées sur des souris afin de déterminer le pouvoir cancérogène du béta-HCH. Dans l'une d'elles, on a administré pendant 110 semaines une dose de 100 mg/kg de nourriture et l'on a observé une hyperplasie du tissu hépatique et une hypertrophie de cet organe. Il y avait également augmentation des tumeurs bénignes et malignes. Dans une autre étude, où la dose administrée était de 500 mg/kg de nourriture pendant une période de 24 semaines, aucune tumeur n'a été observée.

Des études au cours desquelles des rats ont reçu des mélanges de béta-HCH et de biphényles polychlorés donnent à penser que le béta-HCH aurait un effet promoteur.

A la dose de 300 mg/kg de nourriture, le béta-HCH a provoqué une altération sensible de plusieurs des fonctions du système immunitaire en l'espace d'un mois chez la souris.

2.7 Effets sur l'homme

L'examen de travailleurs d'une usine produisant du lindane, exposés à cette substance pendant 7,2 années (en moyenne géométrique, avec des limites de 1 à 30 ans), a permis de conclure que l'exposition professionelle au HCH ne produisait pas de signes d'une atteinte neurologique ni d'une perturbation des fonctions neuromusculaires.

CONCLUSIONS ET RECOMMANDATIONS EN VUE DE LA PROTECTION DE LA SANTE HUMAINE ET DE L'ENVIRONNEMENT (ALPHA- ET BETA-HEXACHLOROCYCLOHEXANES)

1. Conclusions

On ne peut pas comparer les effets nocifs potentiels de l'alpha- et du béta-hexachlorocyclohexane sur l'homme et l'environnement à leurs avantages éventuels, étant donné que ces produits n'ont aucune action insecticide. Leur présence dans l'environnement est donc fort préoccupante. Dans ces conditions, l'usage de produits à base d'HCH technique contenant de fortes concentrations d'alpha- et de béta-HCH n'est en aucun cas justifié.

1.1 Population générale

L'alpha- et le béta-HCH circulent dans l'environnement et sont présents dans les chaînes alimentaires. Il existe donc un risque permanent d'exposition humaine. Cette exposition est faible et devrait lentement diminuer dans les années à venir. Dans ces conditions, il n'y a pas lieu de s'inquiéter sérieusement pour la santé de la population dans son ensemble.

1.2 Sous-groupes de population exposés à un risque particulier

La concentration de l'alpha-HCH dans le lait maternel est faible.

On peut se préoccuper de l'exposition des nourrissons au béta-HCH actuellement présent dans le lait maternel mais il faut malgré tout continuer à encourager l'allaitement maternel.

Il faut cependant faire un maximum d'efforts pour réduire l'exposition par voie alimentaire ou autre à ces isomères. Une moindre exposition d'origine alimentaire à ces substances devrait entraîner une diminution de la teneur du lait maternel en alpha- et béta-HCH.

Conclusions et Recommandations

1.3 Exposition professionnelle

Dans la mesure où elles observent les précautions recommandées en vue réduire au minimum l'exposition à l'alpha- et au béta-HCH, les personnes employées à la fabrication du lindane ne courent pas de risque particulier.

1.4 Effets sur l'environnement

A part le cas de décharge dans le milieu aquatique, rien n'indique que la présence d'alpha- et de béta-HCH dans l'environnement constitue une menace particulière pour la faune et la flore.

2. Recommandations pour la protection de la santé humaine et de l'environnement

a) Afin de réduire au minimum la pollution de l'environnement par l'alpha- et le béta-HCH, il faut utiliser du lindane (> de 99% de gamma-HCH) à la place de l'HCH technique.

b) Pour éviter la pollution de l'environnement par l'alpha- et le béta-HCH, les sous-produits et les effluents issus de la fabrication du lindane doivent être évacués de façon convenable et il faut en particulier éviter la contamination des eaux et du sol.

c) Il faut poursuivre la surveillance de l'alpha- et du béta-HCH dans les denrées alimentaires. Il est essentiel d'instituer un mécanisme par lequel seront fixées des doses limites acceptables sur le plan international pour l'alpha- et le béta-HCH.

d) Il faut poursuivre la surveillance de l'apport quotidien d'alpha- et de béta-HCH et continuer à en contrôler les concentrations dans le lait maternel.

RECHERCHES A EFFECTUER (ALPHA- ET BETA-HEXACHLOROCYCLOHEXANES)

Les études expérimentales suivantes sont nécessaires pour permettre une meilleure évaluation des dangers que représentent l'alpha- et le béta-HCH:

- études de mutagénicité portant en particulier sur les chromosomes;

- études de reproduction, études de foetotoxicité et de tératogénicité;

- études pharmacocinétiques et toxicocinétiques;

- études de cancérogénicité;

- études de neurotoxicité;

- surveillance des populations à risque.

RESUMEN Y EVALUACION

1. Alpha-hexaclorociclohexano

1.1 Propiedades generales

El alpha-hexaclorociclohexano (alpha-HCH) es uno de los principales subproductos (65-70%) de la fabricación del lindano (> 99% gamma-HCH). Su solubilidad en agua es baja, pero es muy soluble en disolventes orgánicos como la acetona, el cloroformo y el xileno. Es una sustancia sólida con baja presión de vapor. El coeficiente de partición n-octanol/agua (log P_{oa}) es 3,82. Se trata de un contaminante ambiental.

El alpha-HCH puede determinarse por separado de los otros isómeros mediante cromatografía de gases con detección de captura electrónica y otros métodos, tras la extracción por partición líquido/líquido y la purificación en cromatografía de columna.

1.2 Transporte, distribución y transformación en el medio ambiente

La biodegradación y la degradación abiótica (decloración) por irradiación ultravioleta tienen lugar en el medio ambiente y producen, respectivamente, delta-3,4,5,6-tetraclorohexeno y pentaclorociclohexeno. Este proceso de degradación es más lento que en el caso del lindano. La persistencia del alpha-HCH en el suelo depende de factores ambientales como la acción de los microorganismos, el contenido de materia orgánica y la codestilación y la evaporación a partir de los suelos. No se produce isomerización del lindano a alpha-HCH.

En los microorganismos se produce una bioconcentración rápida (el factor de bioconcentración es igual a 1500-2700 en peso seco, o aproximadamente 12 000 en lípidos al cabo de 30 minutos), invertebrados (60-2750 (peso seco) o > 8000 (lípidos) al cabo de 24-72 h), y peces (313-1216 al cabo de 4-28 días; hasta 50 000 en el río Elba). No obstante, la biotransformación y la eliminación también son relativamente rápidas en esos organismos (de 15 minutos a 72 h).

1.3 Niveles en el medio ambiente y exposición humana

El alpha-HCH se encuentra en el aire oceánico con una concentración de 0,02-1,5 ng/m^3. En el Canadá, se encontró en el agua de lluvia con una concentración de 1-40 ng/litro, pero sólo se detectaron indicios en la nieve.

Durante el periodo 1969-1974, se encontraron en el río Rin y sus afluentes niveles de alpha-HCH de 0,01-2,7 μg por litro, pero últimamente los niveles han sido inferiores a 0,1 μg/litro. En el río Elba, los niveles disminuyeron desde un promedio de 0,023 mg/litro en 1981 hasta menos de 0,012 μg/litro en 1988. En 1966 se encontró que ciertos ríos del Reino Unido contenían 0,001-0,43 μg por litro. Se ha encontrado alpha-HCH en sedimentos de la región norte del mar de Wadden en concentraciones de 0,3 a 1,4 μg/kg (0,002 μg/litro en el agua).

Las concentraciones de alpha-HCH en diferentes especies vegetales de distintos países variaron entre 0,5-2140 μg/kg en peso seco, pero fueron mucho más altos en zonas contaminadas. Incluso en la Antártida se han encontrado niveles que varían entre 0,2 y 1,15 μg/kg.

El alpha-HCH se detecta con regularidad en peces e invertebrados acuáticos, así como en patos, garzas y lechuzas. En renos y alces de Idaho, que viven en zonas en las que el uso de plaguicidas es prácticamente insignificante, se encontraron niveles medios de alpha-HCH de aproximadamente 70-80 μg/kg en la grasa subcutánea. El tejido adiposo de los osos polares del Canadá contenía 0,3-0,87 mg de alpha-HCH/kg (en grasa).

En varios países se han analizado importantes alimentos en busca de alpha-HCH. Las concentraciones, principalmente en alimentos que contienen grasas, variaron hasta un máximo de 0,05 mg/kg de producto, salvo en la leche y los productos lácteos (hasta 0,22 mg/kg) y en el pescado y en preparaciones de carne (hasta 0,5 mg/kg en grasa). Se ha observado una ligera disminución con los años.

Los alimentos son la principal fuente de exposición de la población general al alpha-HCH. En estudios de la dieta total realizados en los Países Bajos y en el Reino Unido, se encontraron concentraciones medias de 0,01 y 0,002-0,003 mg/kg de alimento, respectivamente. Los datos procedentes del Reino Unido indican una tendencia decreciente desde 1967. En los EE.UU., la ingesta diaria media de alpha-HCH fue de 0,009-0,025 µg/kg de peso corporal durante el periodo 1977-1979, y de 0,003-0,016 µg/kg de peso corporal durante el periodo 1982-1984.

En unos pocos países, se ha determinado la concentración de alpha-HCH en la sangre, el suero o el plasma humanos. La concentración promedio (mediana en algunos casos) fue < 0,1 µg/litro (desde niveles no detectables hasta 0,6 µg/litro). En un país, no obstante, se notificó una concentración media de 3,5 (margen 0,1-15,0) µg por litro. Se detectó alpha-HCH en aproximadamente la tercera parte de las muestras de sangre.

En el ser humano las concentraciones en el tejido adiposo y la leche que se han comunicado son bajas (respectivamente < 0,01-0,1 y < 0,001-0,04 mg/kg en grasa). Los estudios de la dieta total han revelado niveles diarios de ingesta del orden de 0,01 µg/kg de peso corporal por día o menos. Esas concentraciones están disminuyendo poco a poco con los años.

El alpha-HCH parece ser un contaminante ambiental universal. Las concentraciones están disminuyendo muy despacio, a pesar de las medidas adoptadas para impedir su dispersión en el medio ambiente.

1.4 Cinética y metabolismo

En las ratas, el alpha-HCH se absorbe rápida y casi completamente a partir del tracto gastrointestinal. Después de una inyección intraperitoneal, aproximadamente el 40-80% del alpha-HCH se excretó en la orina y el 5-20% en las heces. En la rata, las concentraciones más elevadas se han encontrado en el hígado, los riñones, la grasa, el cerebro y los músculos; el tejido adiposo constituye un importante depósito. Las concentraciones de alpha-HCH en el hígado de las crías lactantes duplicaron las observadas en el hígado de las madres. En la rata, los cocientes cerebro-sangre y grasa de depósito-sangre fueron de 120:1 y 397:1, respectivamente.

La biotransformación del alpha-HCH en la rata entraña la decloración. El principal metabolito urinario es el 2,4,6-triclorofenol; entre otros metabolitos identificados figuran el 1,2,4-, 2,3,4-, y 2,4,5-triclorofenol y el 2,3,4,5- y 2,3,4,6-tetraclorofenol. En el riñón de rata y también en estudios in vitro en hígado de pollo se ha encontrado 1,3,4,5,6-pentaclorociclohex-1-eno. En el hígado se forma un conjugado de glutatión.

En la rata, la semivida de eliminación de la sustancia presente en del depósito graso es de 6,9 días en la hembra y 1,6 días en el macho.

1.5 Efectos en los organismos del medio ambiente

El alpha-HCH tiene baja toxicidad para las algas, siendo por lo general 2 mg/litro el nivel sin efectos observados.

En un estudio a largo plazo, *Daphnia magna* mostró un nivel sin efectos observados de 0,05 mg/litro. El alpha-HCH es moderadamente tóxico para los invertebrados y los peces. Los valores de la $C(E)L_{50}$ aguda para esos organismos son del orden de 1 mg/litro. En estudios a corto plazo con Lebistes reticulatus y Oryzia latipes se observó que 0,8 mg/litro no ejercían efecto alguno.

En estudios de tres meses de duración con *Salmo gairdneri* con dosis de 10-1250 mg/kg de dieta no se observaron efectos en la mortalidad, la conducta, el crecimiento ni las actividades enzimáticas del hígado y el cerebro.

En estudios a corto y a largo plazo con un gasterópodo (*Lymnea stagnalis*) se observó una CE_{50} (basada en la mortalidad y la inmovilización) de 1200 µg/litro. La inhibición de la producción de huevos se produjo con una concentración de 250 µg/litro. Con 65 µg/litro se observó una reducción del 50% en la reproductividad general.

No se dispone de datos sobre los efectos en las poblaciones y los ecosistemas.

1.6 Efectos en animales de experimentación y sistemas de ensayo in vitro

Los valores de la DL_{50} aguda por vía oral en ratones se encuentran entre 1000-4000 y en ratas entre 500 y 4670 mg/kg de peso corporal. Los signos de envenenamiento coinciden principalmente con los de la estimulación del sistema nervioso central.

En un estudio de 90 días de duración en ratas se observó depresión del crecimiento con una concentración de 250 mg/kg de dieta. Los cambios histológicos y enzimáticos en el hígado indicaron inducción enzimática con 50 mg/kg o más. Con esas dosis se observaron también signos de inmunosupresión. Ya se observó aumento del peso hepático con 10 mg/kg de dieta (equivalente a 0,5 mg/kg de peso corporal). El nivel sin efectos adversos observados resultó en este estudio ser 2 mg/kg de dieta (equivalente a 0,1 mg/kg de peso corporal al día).

No se han comunicado estudios adecuados a largo plazo de toxicidad ni estudios de reproducción y teratogenicidad.

Los estudios realizados con diversas cepas de *Salmonella typhimurium* no dieron prueba alguna de mutagenicidad ni con activación metabólica ni sin ella. Los ensayos realizados con *Saccharomyces cerevisiae* también dieron resultado negativo, pero un ensayo de síntesis no programada de ADN en hepatocitos de rata *in vitro* dio resultados ambiguos.

Se ha intentado determinar el potencial carcinogénico en ratones y ratas con dosis de 100 a 600 mg/kg de dieta. En estudios realizados en ratones se encontraron nódulos hiperplásicos y/o adenomas hepatocelulares. En un estudio los niveles de administración excedieron la dosis máxima tolerada. En dos estudios en ratones y uno en ratas, en los que se administraron hasta 160 mg/kg de dieta a ratones y 640 mg/kg de dieta a ratas, no se observó aumento alguno en la incidencia de tumores.

Los resultados de los estudios sobre la iniciación-promoción y el modo de acción, y los estudios de mutagenicidad indican que la tumorigenicidad inducida por el alpha-HCH observada en ratones tiene un mecanismo no genético.

Se ha demostrado que el alpha-HCH provoca un aumento neto de la actividad de los enzimas hepáticos incluso con 5 mg/kg de dieta (equivalente a 0,25 mg/kg de peso corporal). Una dosis de 2 mg/kg de peso corporal no afectó la desmetilación de la aminopirina ni el contenido de ADN en el hígado.

1.7 Efectos en el ser humano

Cuando se examinó a trabajadores de una fábrica de producción de lindano, con una exposición media geométrica de 7,2 años (1-30), se concluyó que la exposición profesional al HCH no induce síntomas de trastornos neurales ni perturbaciones de la "función neuromuscular".

RESUMEN Y EVALUACION

2. Beta-hexaclorociclohexano

2.1 Propiedades generales

El beta-hexaclorociclohexano (beta-HCH) es un subproducto (7-10%) de la fabricación del lindano (> 99% gamma-HCH). Su solubilidad en agua es baja, pero es muy soluble en disolventes orgánicos como la acetona, el ciclohexano y el xileno. Es un sólido con una baja presión de vapor. El coeficiente de partición n-octanol/agua (log P_{oa}) es 3,80. Es un contaminante ambiental.

El beta-HCH puede determinarse por separado de los otros isómeros mediante cromatografía de gases con detección de captura electrónica y otros métodos tras la extracción por partición líquido/líquido y la purificación en cromatografía de columna.

2.2 Transporte, distribución y transformación en el medio ambiente

La biodegradación y la degradación abiótica (decloración) por irradiación ultravioleta tienen lugar en el medio ambiente y producen pentaclorociclohexano, pero a una velocidad mucho menor que en el caso del lindano (gamma-HCH).

El beta-HCH es el isómero más persistente del HCH. Su persistencia en el suelo depende de factores ambientales como la acción de los microorganismos, el contenido de materia orgánica y de agua, y la codestilación y la evaporación a partir del suelo.

Dada la persistencia del beta-HCH, tiene lugar una rápida bioconcentración en invertebrados (el factor de bioconcentración es de aproximadamente 125 al cabo de tres días), peces (250-1500 en peso seco o aproximadamente 500 000 veces en lípidos al cabo de 3-10 días), aves y el hombre (aproximadamente 525). La bioconcentración es más elevada y la eliminación más lenta en el caso del beta-HCH que en los otros isómeros del HCH.

2.3 Niveles ambientales y exposición humana

El beta-HCH se encuentra en el aire oceánico con una concentración de 0,004-0,13 ng/m^3.

Hasta 1974, el río Rin y sus afluentes contenían niveles de beta-HCH de 0,14-0,22 µg/litro, pero después los niveles estuvieron siempre por debajo de 0,1 µg por litro. Las muestras tomadas en el río Mosa también contenían < 0,1 µg/litro. En el río Elba, los niveles descendieron desde un promedio de 0,009 hasta 0,004 µg por litro entre 1981 y 1988.

El beta-HCH se ha medido en aves como el gavilán, el cernícalo, el búho, la garza y el colimbo durante varios años y las concentraciones variaron entre 0,1 y 0,3 mg/kg. Se han encontrado hasta 0,87 mg/kg (en grasa) en el hígado y el tejido adiposo del oso polar.

Se han analizado importantes alimentos en algunos países en busca de beta-HCH. Las concentraciones medias, principalmente en alimentos que contienen grasas, variaron entre 0,03 mg/kg (en grasa), pero en los productos lácteos se encontraron niveles de hasta 4 mg/kg (en grasa). En alimentos no grasos, los niveles fueron < 0,005 mg/kg de producto. En general, los niveles están descendiendo lentamente.

Los alimentos son la principal fuente de exposición de la población general al beta-HCH. En estudios de la dieta total en el Reino Unido, se encontraron 0,003, 0,0005, y < 0,0005 mg/kg durante los años 1966/67, 1975/77 y 1981, respectivamente. En los EE.UU., la ingesta diaria media de beta-HCH en 1982-1984 varió entre < 0,1-0,4 ng/kg de peso corporal en distintos grupos de edad.

En varios países, la concentración de beta-HCH se ha determinado en la sangre, el suero o el plasma de la población general. Las concentraciones variaron entre los distintos países y el máximo encontrado fue de 25 µg por litro.

Se han llevado a cabo numerosos estudios para determinar la presencia de beta-HCH en los tejidos adiposos humanos. Las concentraciones encontradas en el Canadá,

Kenya, los Países Bajos, el Reino Unido, y la República Federal de Alemania, variaron hasta 4,4 mg/kg (en grasa). Se encontró que hasta los 50 años se produce un aumento gradual con la edad; en adelante, los niveles disminuyen. Las concentraciones de beta-HCH en los tejidos adiposos son más altas que las de los otros isómeros del HCH, fenómeno que refleja las propiedades acumulativas del beta-HCH. En general no se ha observado una tendencia clara de disminución de las concentraciones de beta-HCH durante el periodo en que se han hecho los estudios. Existe una relación entre las concentraciones en el tejido adiposo y la leche materna y el consumo de productos cárnicos, grasas animales y pescados grasos.

En unos pocos países (Canadá, Países Bajos, Reino Unido y República Federal de Alemania), se ha analizado la leche humana y se han encontrado niveles de beta-HCH entre 0,1 y 0,69 mg/kg (en grasa). Los niveles medidos en la leche de mujeres de zonas rurales parece ser más elevado que en las de zonas urbanas.

Los elevados niveles de beta-HCH que se han encontrado en la leche materna exceden las concentraciones permisibles a título temporal y local. Las concentraciones de beta-HCH en la sangre de lactantes se encuentran entre los mismos límites que las medidas en las madres.

El beta-HCH parece ser un contaminante ambiental universal. Las concentraciones están disminuyendo muy despacio a pesar de las medidas adoptadas para evitar su dispersión en el medio ambiente.

2.4 Cinética y metabolismo

Hasta el 95% del beta-HCH en el tracto gastrointestinal del ratón es absorbido y a continuación se acumula en su mayor parte en el tejido adiposo. La eliminación sigue un mecanismo de dos etapas; durante la primera, la semivida es de 2,5 días y durante la segunda, 18 días.

Después de la absorción, el beta-HCH se distribuye rápidamente al hígado, el cerebro, los riñones y los tejidos adiposos. En la rata, la concentración máxima en el hígado se alcanza al cabo de cuatro días. Con una concentración sanguínea media de 92 μg/litro (pero también con concentraciones de 540 y 2100 μg/litro), los cocientes cerebro-sangre y tejido adiposo-sangre fueron 2:1 y 170:1, respectivamente. Tras el envenenamiento agudo y mortal de un hombre con isómeros de HCH, la concentración de beta-HCH, en relación con la de la sangre, fue de 363 en la grasa, 3 en el cerebro y 15 en el hígado. El beta-HCH atraviesa la barrera hematoencefálica con mucha menos facilidad que los demás isómeros del HCH.

En el ratón, el paso transplacentario de la hembra gestante al feto fue de aproximadamente el 2% de la dosis, pero en la rata se observó un paso del 40%. En la rata, la transferencia de la madre al lactante en la leche fue de aproximadamente el 60% de la dosis.

En la rata, el 70% del beta-HCH se elimina durante 28 días; un tercio de esa cantidad se excreta en la orina. No aparece beta-HCH sin modificar en la orina. El principal metabolito procedente de la cis-deshidrocloración es el 2,4,6-triclorofenol en forma conjugada.

El pretratamiento con beta-HCH altera el metabolismo del lindano en las ratas. Según estudios intraperitoneales realizados en ratones, parece que el beta-HCH se metaboliza con más lentitud que el lindano.

2.5 Efectos en los organismos del medio ambiente

En general, el beta-HCH tiene una toxicidad moderada para las algas, los invertebrados y los peces. Los valores de la DL_{50} aguda para esos organismos son del orden de 1 mg/litro, pero los valores de la CE_{50} son más bajos (0,05-0,5 mg/litro). El nivel sin efectos observados en *Oryzia latipes* y *Poecilia reticulata*, dos peces de agua dulce expuestos durante 1 ó 3 meses, fue de 0,03 mg por litro.

No se dispone de datos sobre los efectos en las poblaciones y los ecosistemas.

2.6 Efectos en animales de experimentación y sistemas de ensayo in vitro

Los valores de DL_{50} aguda por vía oral en ratones y ratas comunicados en 1968 se encontraban entre 1500 y 2000 mg/kg de peso corporal. No obstante, en estudios más recientes se han obtenido valores de 16 g/kg de peso corporal en ratones y 8 g/kg de peso corporal en ratas. Los signos de intoxicación fueron principalmente de origen neural.

En dos estudios en ratones a corto plazo, con dosis de hasta 600 mg/kg de dieta durante 26-32 semanas, se observó un aumento del peso hepático, así como hiperplasia nodular y proliferaciones atípicas en el hígado. En un tercer estudio, la administración de hasta 500 mg/kg de dieta durante 24 semanas no produjo tumores hepáticos ni hiperplasia nodular.

En un estudio a 90 días con ratas a las que se administraron 50 ó 250 mg/kg de dieta se observaron cambios hepáticos, a saber, hipertrofia y proliferación del retículo endoplásmico liso y mayor actividad de los enzimas microsómicas. Con las dosis más altas se produjeron cambios en las gónadas pero éstos estuvieron asociados a modificaciones muy acusadas del peso corporal. Los cambios hormonales asociados a la atrofia gonadal no mostraron un efecto endocrino consecuente. No se observaron efectos adversos con una dosis de 2 mg/kg de dieta (equivalente a 0,1 mg/kg de peso corporal).

En un estudio en ratas a largo plazo (comunicado en 1950), la administración de dosis de 10 mg/kg de dieta (equivalente a 0,5 mg/kg de peso corporal) o superiores produjo dilatación y cambios histológicos en el hígado.

En un estudio de reproducción de ratas en dos generaciones, se observaron los mismos efectos que en el estudio de 90 días. No se observaron efectos con 2 mg/kg de dieta (equivalente a 0,1 mg/kg de peso corporal), pero con una dosis de 10 mg/kg de dieta aumentaron la mortalidad y la infecundidad. En una ampliación de este estudio no se observaron efectos teratogénicos relacionados con el compuesto.

Se ha descrito un ligero efecto "estrogénico". El órgano diana de este efecto era el útero; no se apreciaron efectos claros en los sistemas de control endocrino. No se sabe con seguridad cuál es el mecanismo ni el significado de este efecto.

Los estudios de mutagenicidad comunicados no mostraron aumento alguno en la frecuencia de mutaciones en cepas de *Salmonella typhimurium*. En un análisis *in vivo* de la metafase en médula ósea de ratas se obtuvieron resultados positivos.

Se han llevado a cabo dos estudios en el ratón para determinar el potencial carcinogénico. En uno de los estudios, se administraron 200 mg/kg de dieta durante 110 semanas, y se notificaron dilatación del hígado, cambios hiperplásicos y aumento de tumores tanto benignos como malignos. En el otro estudio, en el que se administraron 500 mg/kg de dieta durante 24 semanas, no se observaron tumores.

En estudios en los que se administró a ratas combinaciones de beta-HCH con bifenilos policlorados se sugirió que el beta-HCH tenía un efecto de promoción.

Con 300 mg/kg de dieta, el beta-HCH provocó cambios significativos en varias funciones inmunitarias en el ratón al cabo de un mes.

2.7 Efectos en el ser humano

Cuando se examinó a trabajadores de una fábrica de producción de lindano, con una exposición media geométrica de 7,2 años (1-30), se concluyó que la exposición profesional al HCH no induce signos de trastornos neurales ni de perturbación de la "función neuromuscular".

CONCLUSIONES Y RECOMENDACIONES PARA LA PROTECCION DE LA SALUD HUMANA Y DEL MEDIO AMBIENTE (ALPHA- Y BETA-HEXACLOROCICLOHEXANOS)

1. Conclusiones

Los efectos adversos potenciales del alpha- y el beta-hexaclorociclohexano (HCH) en el ser humano y el medio ambiente no pueden sopesarse frente a sus beneficios, puesto que estos isómeros no tienen acción insecticida. Su presencia en el medio ambiente es por tanto causa de gran inquietud. En consecuencia, en ningún caso se justifica el uso de productos técnicos del HCH que contengan elevadas concentraciones de alpha- y beta-HCH.

1.1 Población general

El alpha- y el beta-HCH circulan en el medio ambiente y están presentes en las cadenas alimentarias. Así pues, existe un potencial continuo de exposición humana. Esta exposición es baja y se espera que disminuya lentamente en los años por venir. Así pues, no hay motivos de gran inquietud en cuanto a la salud de la población general.

1.2 Subpoblaciones especialmente expuestas

Las concentraciones de alpha-HCH en la leche humana son bajas.

La exposición de lactantes debida a las actuales concentraciones de beta-HCH en la leche materna es preocupante, pero no suficiente para dejar de fomentar la lactancia natural.

No obstante, debe hacerse todo lo posible para disminuir la exposición a esos isómeros por la vía alimentaria y por toda otra vía. Se espera que la menor exposición por la dieta dé como resultado menores niveles de alpha- y beta-HCH en la leche humana.

1.3 Exposición profesional

Mientras se observen las precauciones recomendadas para reducir al mínimo la exposición del personal que trabaja en la fabricación del lindano, el alpha- y el beta-HCH no plantean riesgos para la salud de los operarios.

1.4 Efectos en el medio ambiente

Aparte de los vertidos en el medio acuático, no hay pruebas que sugieran que la presencia de alpha- y beta-HCH en el medio ambiente plantee un riesgo significativo para las poblaciones de seres vivos.

2. Recomendaciones para la protección de la salud humana y el medio ambiente

a) A fin de reducir al mínimo la contaminación ambiental con alpha- y beta-HCH, debe usarse lindano (< 99% gamma-HCH) en lugar de HCH técnico.

b) A fin de evitar la contaminación ambiental con alpha- y beta-HCH, los subproductos y los efluentes de la fabricación del lindano deben evacuarse de modo apropiado, y debe evitarse la contaminación de aguas naturales y del suelo.

c) Debe proseguir la vigilancia del alpha- y del beta-HCH en los alimentos. Es imprescindible poner en marcha un mecanismo para establecer niveles internacionalmente aceptables de alpha- y beta-HCH en los alimentos.

d) Debe proseguir la vigilancia de la ingesta diaria de la población general y de los niveles de alpha- y beta-HCH en la leche materna.

OTRAS INVESTIGACIONES (ALPHA- Y BETA-HEXACLOROCICLOHEXANOS)

Deben hacerse los estudios siguientes para evaluar mejor los riesgos del alpha- y el beta-HCH:

- oestudios de mutagenicidad, especialmente con puntos terminales mutagénicos en los cromosomas;

- oestudios de reproducción y fetotoxicidad/teratogenicidad;

- oestudios farmacocinéticos y toxicocinéticos;

- oestudios de carcinogenicidad;

- oestudios de neurotoxicidad;

- oestudios de vigilancia de poblaciones en riesgo.